Flynn's Outback Angels
Casting the Mantle

Volume I
1901 to World War II

Ivan Rudolph

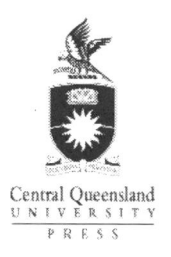

Central Queensland
UNIVERSITY
PRESS

© Ivan Rudolph 2001

This book is copyright. Apart from any fair dealing for the purpose of private study, research, criticism or review, as permitted under the Copyright Act of 1968, no part may be reproduced by any process without written permission. Enquiries should be made to the publisher.

First published in 2001 by
Central Queensland University Press (Outback Books)
PO Box 1615
Rockhampton, Queensland 4700
Phone: (07) 4923 2520
Fax: (07) 4923 2525
email: d.myers@cqu.edu.au
Web: www.outbackbooks.com

National Library of Australia
Cataloguing-in-Publication entry:

Rudolph, Ivan. Flynn's outback angels. Volume 1, Casting the mantle, 1901–World War II
1. Australian Inland Mission. 2. Rural nursing -
Queensland. 3. Nurses - Queensland - Biography. I. Title.

ISBN 1 875998 91 8.

610.734309943

Typeset in 11 on 13 point Berkeley by
Frank Povah at The Busy Boordy, Tenterfield.

Printed and bound by Watson Ferguson & Co., Brisbane.

Cover design: Frank Povah
Front cover: AIM 50th Anniversary Commemorative Stamp issued 5th September 1962. Designed by F.D. Manley, this was the first multicolour stamp to be produced in Australia by the photogravure process. Courtesy National Philatelic Collection, Australia Post, with special thanks to Georgia Cribb and Russell Hick.
Front cover: AIM Nurses at Oodnadatta, SA. Photo courtesy Meg McKay.

Acknowledgements

As I look around my study, I see that I am surrounded by the source material for this book: faxes, photographs, emails, typed accounts, handwritten letters, personal diaries, cassette tapes and notes from telephone conversations. This abundance of material has been graciously supplied by women who served in the bush or by their families. I am sincerely grateful to each and every one of them for their interest and generosity in sharing their personal memories. I have appreciated their support and suggestions and hope they will enjoy the results of our shared labour.

The late Fred McKay and his wife Meg were wonderfully helpful to me with advice, information and encouragement.

I wish to thank David Myers, my publisher at Central Queensland University Press. David has been very encouraging and perceptive. He works extraordinarily long hours, driven by his love for Australia, for the bush and for books.

I am delighted that the ABC recognises John Flynn and his "outback angels" as national icons, and considers their stories worthy of a co-production with CQUP in a determined attempt to reach across Australia. In particular, I thank for their support:

Ross Quinn (Manager of ABC Rockhampton)
Colin Munro (ABC Manager Regional Liaison
   and Resources)
Daniel Jordon (National Manager of ABC Centres)
Stuart Neal (Commissioning Editor ABC Enterprises)

I would like to thank my friends Ruth Glanville and Jeff Coutts for reading the manuscript and offering valuable suggestions and corrections, and Paul Cruice for composing the concise map at the front of the book.

I especially thank Brenda, my wife. Often when I crawl out of bed in the early hours of the morning to write, she asks sleepily "Are you off to your first love now?" Yet despite her concerns about my supposed affection for the computer, which incidentally I hate but can't live without anymore, she gives me a great deal of support and advice. She is involved with the whole process and also does a good job with her initial editing of the material. I could not write without her... or the computer... or her.... or the computer... etc.

I am grateful to Jason, my son, who has helped often and very patiently with my rather perverse computer.

The successful completion of this book, and its companion volume, would not have been possible without the valuable input of all the above people.

Photographic Credits

Most of the photographs have been generously loaned by private individuals. Others have been published by courtesy of the following institutions:

The John Oxley Library, Brisbane;
The Northern Territory Library;
Queensland Museum;
The National Library, Canberra;
Northern Territory Times;
State Library of South Australia

Conversion Table

Approximate metric conversions for the imperial measurements used in this book are given below.

1 foot	0.3 metre	1 mile	1.61 kilometres
1 acre	0.4 hectare	1 gallon	4.55 litres
1 pound (lb)	0.45 kilogram	1 ton	1.02 tonnes

110°Fahrenheit = 43°Celsius   120°Fahrenheit = 49°Celsius

Australian Currency until 1965

1 pound (£) = 20 shillings (s)   1 shilling = 12 pence (d)

When Australia adopted the dollar ($) it was based on 10s. At the time of Federation (1901) £1 would be the equivalent of more than $100 today. However, comparing currency in this way can be misleading. In the early twentieth century, for example, a bicycle could cost £30, more than three months wages for some people.

Contributors

I acknowledge with gratitude the following contributors, along with any inadvertently omitted. Their generous contributions have made these volumes possible. To those who may have been overlooked, my apologies.

Irene Ackland
Jean Ackland
Ann Adams
Elizabeth Aird
Jean Auld
Dulcie Andrew
Jean Ashlowe
Helen Balmain
Alice Barclay
Margaret Bates
Dorothy Beard
Amelia Beckett
William Bett
Ann Blakely
Rosemary Bolton
Irene Brand
David Brooke
Beth Brown
Joan Brown
Elizabeth Burchill
Lillian Clark
Mollie Clark
Beth Clarke
Roy and
    Margaret Cosier
Alaine Crowder
Linda Daly
Shirley Debney
Janet Dickinson
Dulcie Easey
Margaret Easey
Betty Ewin
Helen Ferguson
Raylee Finlen
Margaret Ford
Laurel Frahn
Rachel Frend
Jan Gall
Beth Garrett
Rill Gibson
Arch Grant
Beryl Grant
Colleen Grieve

Pat Grimoldby
Lorna Gwydir
Alice Hall
Dorothy Hargreaves
Joan Harrison
Marion Hawley
Dorothy Herbert
Betty Hildebrand
Billie Hill
Kathleen Holloman
Helen Hooke
Phyllis Hughes
Judith Hunt
Beth Ireland
Mavis Johnson
John Jones
Derek Keene
Phyllis Keifel
Flo Laver
Helen Lawson
Billie Lennon
Marjorie London
Marjorie Longton
Douglas Lyons
Heather McAuley
Enid MacDonald
Helen McFarlane
Beryl McGregor
Elizabeth "Meg" McKay
Fred McKay
Elspeth McKay
Judith McKay
Lyn McKay
Eula McLean
Bernice McLeod
Shirley McNaught
Eunice Mann
Alan Matthews
Jennifer Meyenn
Peter Miethke
Ronda Mitchell
Clive and
    Margaret Morey

John Morley
Phil Morton
June Mott
Joy Motter
Angela Neuhaus
Suzanne Nilon
Mary Nugent
Chris Patt
Ruth Paynter
George and
    Phyllis Keifel
Joy Ramsay
Grace Reid
Fay Richardson
Roz Rose
Nancy Rose
Maisie Ross
Chris Rowe
Nan Schrivener
Beryl Scott
Regine Searle
Helen Seers
Olive Shute
Jean Smith
Ron and
    Audrey Sparks
Beth Symonds
Robyn Taylor
Elwyn Tegel
Betty Timmins
Helen Tolcher
Donna Vanclay
Lois Walker
Margaret Wells
John Weymouth
Catherine Wheatley
Jean Whimp
Jean Whitla
Betty White
Ruth White
Brenda Wilson
Rosemary Young
Wendy Young

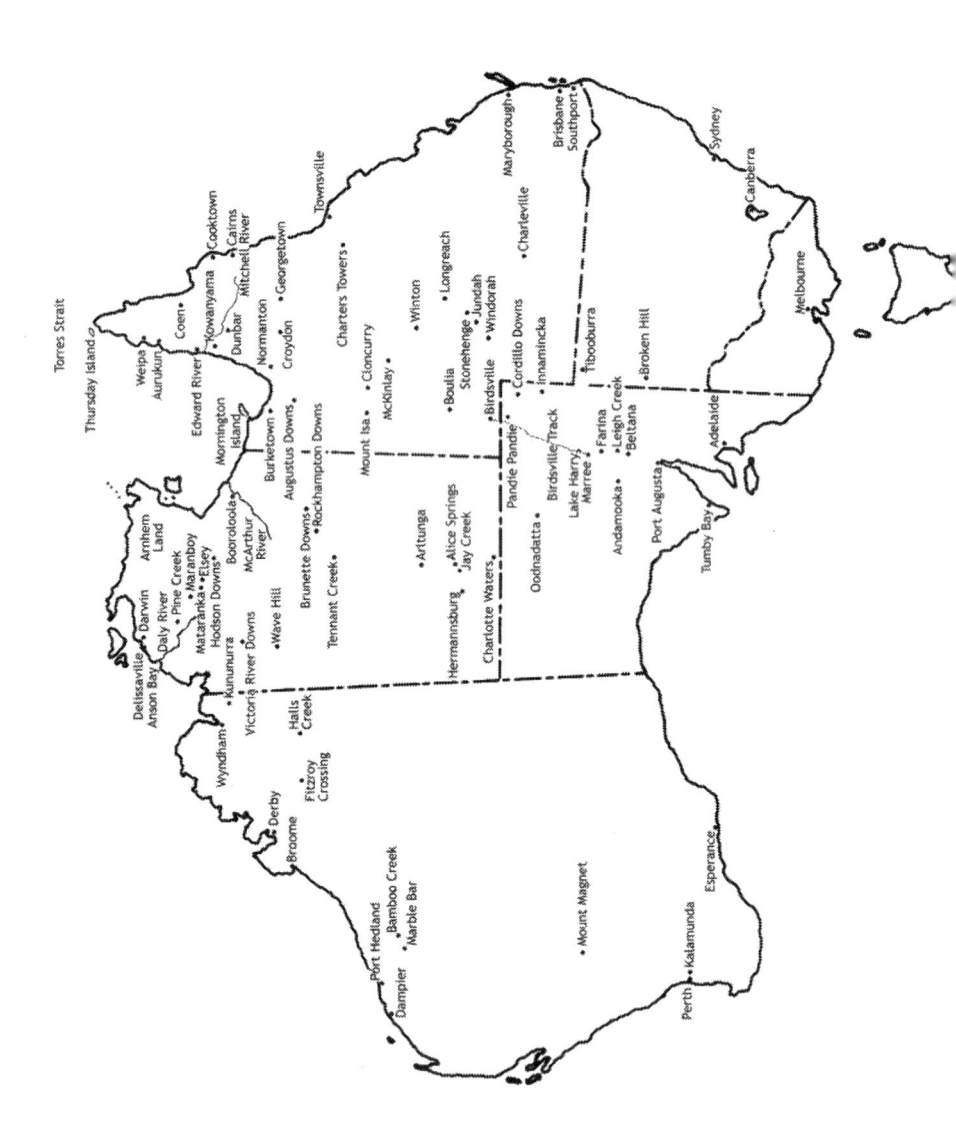

Casting the mantle over Australia's outback

Introduction

While researching for my earlier book on the great John Flynn, it struck me that the role women played in establishing and maintaining his "Mantle of Safety" over the Australian Inland had never been given sufficient credit. A nurse I know, who had worked for Flynn, clapped her hands when I told her that I would like to write a book about this and said, "About time!"

The central reason that Flynn sought the medical and social cooperation of women is often misunderstood. Let me try to clarify this pivotal point, as appreciation of his methodology is impossible until his vision is understood.

Flynn did want to bring to the bush medical help and thereby also freedom from fear—his nurses, cottage hospitals and Flying Doctors all speak of that.

But they were not his main purpose.

Flynn did want to promote a close and caring community in the outback, and his Patrol Padres and the social work of his nurses all contributed.

But that was not his main purpose.

Flynn did want to break down the isolation and find how to allow the "dumb bush to speak", and his wireless network brought about a social revolution.

But that was not his main purpose.

None of the above was the fundamental reason for Flynn's work in the bush.

The wireless network, Flying Doctors and nursing services together formed his famous Mantle of Safety that protected the isolated areas of Australia. But even the Mantle of Safety was not Flynn's primary purpose. In fact, Flynn's Christian mission, the Australian Inland Mission (AIM), had been ministering to the Inland for a number of years before the concept of a Mantle of Safety was even formulated.

What, then, was Flynn's fundamental purpose regarding the Inland? And why did it involve women?

Flynn stated unequivocally that: "The very presence of women in increasing numbers in the bush would 'sweeten' life there."

This was his brilliant strategy for solving the horrendous moral and spiritual problems outlined in the letter written to him by Jessie Litchfield in 1909! That same letter represented his calling and the role that women could play became the inspiration for his missionary endeavours. [It is quoted in full later, in Jessie's biography.]

And that is why Flynn sought out and obtained the help of so many women, and why he did all he could to encourage women to live in the outback, and why the Mantle of Safety was devised.

The Mantle of Safety was not an end in itself, only the means to an end. Its purpose, and everything else Flynn did, was to promote the presence of women in the bush because they would sweeten life there.

For those who would disagree, I refer you to Flynn's own writings on the matter and his 1912 and 1914 reports to the General Assembly of the Presbyterian Church. Just one quote from his seminal 1912 report, from which the AIM and his whole later ministry evolved, will illustrate this point:

> The first thing to do in any effort to uplift the tone of bush life is to give women a sense of security; in other words, to make childbearing comparatively safe at the outposts. Then brave men will not hesitate to lead partners further back, and the presence of women and white children in greater numbers will sweeten the whole life.

How better, to achieve this end, than to have women go out into the bush as part of his missionary work? And to have those women who were already there networking with his mission?

Nor did he change this view even when he lost nurses through marriage to Inlanders. A decade later he wrote: "Sister Elsie King, after returning to her people for a time, will return to the Territory and be married to one of its hard-toiling citizens. You probably know that one of our former nurses of Maranboy is now Mrs Harold Giles of Bonrook, near Pine Creek. Unofficially we are rather gratified at these sequels, which should mean more permanent gains to the land we strive to serve."

A favourite saying of his was, "Good women make good men."

In 1934 he wrote: "We strive to make the Lonely Lands reasonably happy and safe for children and women, the climax of our many efforts for Christ and Continent. No women, no future."

Consequently he was way ahead of his time in his comprehensive involvement of women in his ministry. The church of the day was very much a man's world and women played a relatively low-key role. But right from the start, women needed to be pivotal in Flynn's work if his dreams were to be realised.

Men of the bush, and even the media, agreed with Flynn's approach. The *Northern Territory Times* editorialised this view as early as 1917 when commending the work done in Flynn's cottage hospital at Maranboy:

> The presence of the hospital and its conveniences has encouraged the men to bring their womenfolk to the settlement, and the result is an immense improvement in the comfort and social conditions of this pioneer township. With no fear of sickness, the womenfolk are going to Maranboy, and there is no greater hope for the field than in this progress.

Nor was it only men who shared this opinion; women embraced it as well. No less a person than Lady Aspley paid this tribute to the Sisters at Wimmera Home, one of Flynn's cottage hospitals in the Territory, after she visited it in 1925:

> The advent of two nurses is an inestimable boon and an encouragement to white women to follow their husbands and fathers into the bush. The greatest difficulty hitherto has been to get the women to live in the Inland of the Northern Territory, and one of the chief reasons up to now has been the entire lack of medical attention, so that the Australian Inland Mission is doing a great practical work for the development of the Northern Territory by making it possible for a married man to take his wife to live there on these lonely stations. Moreover, the social addition of two charming, unmarried white women fresh from town is enormously appreciated by every man in the Territory, who sometimes never sees a white woman from one year's end to another.

And how did nurses who married Inlanders, and stayed there to raise families, envision their contribution? Sister Norma Cross (Fitzroy Crossing 1943–44) sees it this way:

> Dr Flynn's main aim was to provide some security and companionship to white women in the outback, not just to those already there, so that men would feel more confident in bringing back a bride.
>
> I married a local bachelor and Quanbun [cattle station] became my home, until our elder son took over. He also married an AIM Sister! Dr Flynn would have been pleased!

Perhaps this is an understatement; I am sure Flynn would have been delighted.

The Title

Some may say that the title *Flynn's Outback Angels* is inappropriate. "The boys at the Cairns Base and I had a good laugh about the idea of 'Flynn's Angels'; I was no angel," was a typical comment made to me.

In my defence, the title is not exclusively mine; it came out of the bush itself. For example, Sister Bett was known widely as "The Little Angel of the North" and Flying Doctor Jean White was written up as "The Angel of the Gulf Country". Even that crusty old bushman, Lou Reese, wrote to Flynn regarding two nurses he had watched in action while taking them to Birdsville: "If ever angels came to earth, I would say these are two."

Perhaps it is in what they do rather than who they are that has caused these women to be described as angels? Perhaps desperately sick people associated their white uniforms and their solace with angels?

I close my case by quoting in full a letter sent to Sisters Herd and Dunlop when they left Maranboy (1922):

> To the Angels of the Bush.
> Dear Angels,
> I am enclosing a cheque as an appreciation from Roper Valley, Nutwood, Mataranke and old Dan Dillon, of your wonderful goodness and kindness to all bush folk. We want you to buy

some little token of remembrance when you reach Brisbane, and we all wish you both every happiness and all sorts of luck wherever you go.

Goodbye, dear girls. God be with you always.
Yours sincerely,
Arthur Morrice.

The Scope

When I told Arch Grant six years ago over the telephone that I intended to write about the women who had helped to implement Flynn's vision, he chuckled and commented: "Rather you than me." Why, I wondered? Arch was one of Flynn's prominent Patrol Padres and had written several books himself; so why was he hesitant about a book to recognise the input that women had made?

As I began research for this book six years ago, I started to comprehend what Arch had meant—the topic was too huge. There had been hundreds of women with great stories who all deserved recognition. It was impossible to do the subject justice.

I might have abandoned the concept had not Fred McKay, Betty Ewin, Ron Sparks, Clive Morey, Jean Auld, Jean Whimp and others been so enthusiastic and helpful. And my letters soliciting information produced a terrific response from many of that great band of women who have served in the Inland.

After much thought, I accepted that it was not possible for me to do a thorough historical account. Rather, I decided, I would produce a representative book, one that sampled what was done and what it was like. Of course, much of the material that had been sent to me by the women, good material that deserved publishing, would be left out. That was disappointing but unavoidable. The material sent to me has not been wasted, though, because all of it has given me a feel for what was involved even if it is not quoted directly.

What to put in and what to leave out became the next question. I decided not to feature women who have been written about extensively already, in the main, but rather to break lots of new ground. However, I will point readers to relevant books regarding great women such as Sister Latto Bett, Mona Henry, Elizabeth Burchill, Margaret Ford and Robin Miller. Each of them deserves a chapter written about her, but will only be mentioned briefly. But even after I had cut out much material, I could see two books were needed.

The first covers, loosely, up to the Second World War and deals mainly with heroic nursing, while the second deals with those who did their most significant work after the war and in it we meet we meet women Flying Doctors, vets, dentists, pilots, social workers, Flight Sisters and educationalists—leading to the School of the Air. There was an explosion in the roles that women played in the outback following the Second World War.

I have structured the books more-or-less chronologically, although many of the lives overlapped.

Finally, the books are designed as sequels to *John Flynn*, which gives the wider context and overall development of the Mantle of Safety within which these women played such a significant role. The three books thereby form a set and each needs the others for the full picture to be grasped.

Contents

	Acknowledgements	iii
	Conversion Table	iv
	List of Contributors	v
	Introduction	vii
1.	The Brave Pioneer—Jeannie Gunn	1
2.	Snippets About Pioneering Women and the Conditions They faced	19
3.	The Inspiration—Jessie Litchfield	26
4.	Nurses Without Hospitals—Jean Finlayson and Minnie Kinnear	52
5.	Snippets of Journeys	88
6.	Birdsville Needs a Hospital—Grace Francis	93
7.	Flynn's Early Nurses in Snapshot	115
8.	Flynn's Friends—The Inglis Sisters	127
9.	Diaries and Romance at Alice Springs	150
10.	Territorian Heroes—Ruth Heathcock and Elsie Jones	162
11.	They Also Served—Jean Flynn and Others	187
12.	Flynn's First Woman Flying Doctor—Jean White	195

1

The Brave Pioneer—Jeannie Gunn

"You look fine now, dear. Go and sit on the green box," Jeannie's mother instructed her and Jeannie went to join the others already sitting there in a line. There were six children, four girls and two boys, and dressing them to go to church in the fussy clothing of the 1870s took time. However, their father was Reverend Thomas Taylor and it would not have done for the children to look anything less than perfect in church. Jeannie and her siblings hated sitting still, so much so that their mother turned "go and sit on the green box" into the family punishment for minor misdemeanours, the length of time spent there being related to the degree of offence. The children would engage in lively conversation while they sat there.

"You couldn't have! You couldn't have!"

"Yes, I did remember it too!"

"Mother, Jeannie says she remembers something that happened before she was born. Tell her she couldn't have."

"I did too. I was watching. You see that pretty dust in that shaft of sunshine? Well, I was the dust blowing around the room."

Her mother stopped combing hair and turned to look thoughtfully at Jeannie. She did not reprimand her for lying because she understood childish fantasies. What arrested her, and not for the first time, was Jeannie's unusual power of description, "I was the dust blowing around the room" was not the level of expression you would expect from a young child. How might this gifting be used, she wondered?

After church one day Jeannie told her mother in great excitement, "I know what I want to be when I grow up. I belong to Jesus and he healed people, so I want to be a medical missionary."

Mrs Taylor paused thoughtfully before she replied. This was an era when there were no openings for girls to train in the medical field. Besides, they were a poor family and could not

1

afford formal schooling for more than the two eldest in the family, so she would be schooling Jeannie at home. But she did not want to dampen the little sprite's enthusiasm, so she said, "That's very nice, Jeannie. Perhaps you will play a part in healing people, their souls as well as their bodies like Jesus did, but personally I think you will do whatever falls into your lap."

This expression captured Jeannie's attention and she decided she would trust God to bring along whatever he wanted for her lap. Not that she had a very big lap, being the tiniest in her family, but God would know just how much it could hold.

Jeannie was chosen by her friends whenever a game required someone small and she displayed both agility and pluck. Sometimes she would hang precariously by a rope over the side of their home to gather up imaginary flowers, in her mind's eye the edelweiss growing on alpine slopes. Her suppleness and enjoyment of dance developed into a love for gymnastics and she bought and used Indian clubs and dumb-bells. To the amusement of her siblings, she developed an early morning workout routine that she stuck to faithfully over the years.

Jeannie and her sisters had a problem: what to do with their lives? They had no desire to enter domestic service, nor did they want to flutter their eyelashes at every man who appeared. They were bright and independent. If love and marriage came along that would be all very well but they refused to enter the social round to court it. Openings for women in the 1880s were strictly limited, however, especially for those whose education had been curtailed. Their mother's teaching had been good ("The best education of all," Jeannie often said) and they had all matriculated and could have gone on to university had money been available, but it wasn't. So the sisters gathered to have a serious discussion. Jeannie, born in 1870, was the youngest.

"We should set up a school here, at our home. We have plenty of room and between us could teach every subject."

"Yes, and I'll teach gymnastics too," Jeannie cut in enthusiastically.

And so it was decided, the children would set up and run a school from their home.

Realising they would be judged harshly, they were very professional and thorough in their approach. Their prospectus offered a wide variety of subjects, from kindergarten to matriculation. What should they call their school? They reversed their surname, Taylor, and called it "Rolyat".

Rolyat operated from 1889 to 1896, after which Jeannie continued as a visiting teacher in local schools. One of her pupils wrote later that "an outing with Miss Taylor was as exciting as setting off for the moon" because of Jeannie's sense of fun and adventure, which was allied to penetrating observations that she made about life around them as they journeyed along. And when she walked, she tripped along lightly with energy and verve.

Jeannie was musical and loved drama and concerts. When attending the theatre one night in 1901, the horses backed and she slipped forwards as she tried to step out of the buggy. A nearby stranger reacted quickly, dashed forward and caught her as she fell, then was surprised at how light she felt in his arms. His name was Aeneas Gunn and it was the start of a giddy romance.

She discovered that Aeneas, a decade her senior, was an unusual person. He had a sensitive, artistic nature and was a librarian who wrote stories and poetry. He also sketched, both landscapes and people, and these were of a good standard. She found great affinity with this side of his nature, and also with his sense of fun and his Christian convictions. Like her, he had grown up in a minister's home, his father being the Reverend Peter Gunn who had ridden throughout Victoria to hold meetings wherever possible, even in open fields, and who had preached to country folk in both English and Gaelic.

But there was another side of Aeneas' nature with which Jeannie was unfamiliar. He was a bushman who had spent a decade droving cattle in the wild North. Amongst other enterprises, he had worked alongside the renowned Joseph Bradshaw of "Bradshaw's Run" and had helped to establish Victoria River Downs station, the largest in the world at that time. His yearning for the wide-open spaces was making him restless.

Aeneas passed her copies of a series of articles he had written years before in the *Melbourne Leader* regarding an interesting journey he had made in 1891 for Joseph Bradshaw, accompanying Mary Jane Bradshaw to her wealthy husband's property in the Top End. The articles read like an adventure story until they finally made it, despite the heat turning them into "twelve roasting human beings". In these articles Aeneas had not glossed over the extraordinary difficulties faced by a woman of culture trying to adapt to the rigours of the Territory. How had the experiment ended? Despite all the effort, Mary Jane had returned to Melbourne shortly afterwards and never again lived in the North, though remaining married to Joseph Bradshaw. Aeneas had written generously of the departing Mary Jane:

> Mrs Bradshaw leaves for Derby. She has shown no little heroism in going to such an out of the way corner of the funny old round world at all and had, after a fair trial of it, decided that she and life at Marigui could not agree. Tent life in the Australian tropics, even during an ordinary summer and in the most favourable circumstances, has not a great many features to recommend it to a lady... Mrs Bradshaw must have found the absence of congenial feminine society a sore trial and a sufficient reason for shaking the dust of Marigui off her feet.

He and Jeannie discussed these articles in depth, each saying what they felt about them and the issues faced by a woman of culture from the South trying to adapt to the lifestyle and difficulties of the North. Aeneas said he had understood Mary Jane's decision to leave despite the enormous difficulties he had to overcome taking her there. Jeannie said she felt that true love should be able to conquer great trials, including that of living in the Territory without the company of other women.

Jeannie soon discovered this had not been a discussion without another motive. Aeneas dropped a bombshell one evening. He told her that he wanted to return to the Top End, as manager of Elsey station, a significant property of more than a million acres. It was on the Roper River near Katherine in the Territory. He had fallen in love with her and wanted her to come with him as his wife. Having pictured already what would be involved, she was undaunted and accepted at once.

It is at this point, as they journeyed to Elsey in 1901, that readers of Jeannie's bush classic *We Of The Never-Never* first meet the newly-weds.

How might this diminutive (152 cm) woman, raised in the sheltered suburbs of Melbourne, adjust to the rigours of life in the bush?

Firstly, she was very determined. The men at Elsey did not want her on the cattle property as they thought she would spoil their lifestyle and a war of telegrams resulted when the couple reached Darwin. The men at Elsey were trying to discourage her from coming. The telegrams were not confidential and the Darwinites sniggered at the situation. The womenfolk also tried to dissuade Jeannie from going further, giving examples of the difficulties of life in the bush. Jeannie firmly repeated her resolve to proceed regardless.

Her gustiness and physical fitness were vital during their gruelling trip to Elsey. She had to dangle on a wire and be pulled over a swollen river, the Fergusson, while the men yelled encouragement. When she sagged dangerously close to the rushing waters, Mac, the "Head Stockman", yanked too hard and she went shooting up into the air—yet she remained cool and unflustered. It was fortunate that she had climbed ropes as a child, hanging out of trees and down the sides of their home. This time it was not children but hardened bushmen who watched her swinging aloft. They said little but began to think that perhaps she was a "good un" after all. This impression was heightened when she crossed the swollen Edith in a tiny rowing boat, and the King at full gallop in the buckboard. They watched as she swam her horse across smaller creeks with her husband taking the reins. Her horse would drift and stumble before clambering up the other bank, but she never panicked. That she was a keen and expert horsewoman was obvious, but it was her courage that was most important to them. Without courage she would have been a liability.

Along with an unwelcoming work force, other problems met Jeannie at Elsey. She had hoped for a "commodious homestead" fitting for the manager of over a million acres, but the cyclone of

1897 had blown it to bits and it had been partially rebuilt into "verandas and promises". There was only one room completed in the shell, their bedroom. The rest was open to the elements although covered by a corrugated-iron roof. Muddy dog prints wandered up the walls and ceiling because they had not been removed from the planks when the house had been rebuilt. Once again, she impressed the men with her bright acceptance of the conditions and her optimism that the home could be put in order quickly. Aeneas, now known as the "Maluka", warned her that planks to do the job "grow in trees in these parts and have to be coaxed out with a saw", not to mention the seasoning process that had to follow. Jeannie still refused to be discouraged. She rode in the forest and chose trees from which the planks for her home were sawn.

Meanwhile she got on with being a housewife as well as an extra hand on the property.

With charm and sensitivity, she gradually won the respect of the work force, then their affection. Though slowly given, it was never revoked. The last to succumb was the "Quiet Stockman", Jack McLeod, a Scot who had a deep-seated mistrust of women because, he felt, they didn't know anything about the bush and asked too many questions anyway. Jeannie observed that when the men took out books to read in the evenings by the firelight, Jack never turned the page, so she surmised that he could not read but was too embarrassed to say so. Selecting her moment carefully so as not to increase his discomfort at his lack of education, Jeannie taught him to read—and another lifelong friendship was born. Some years later, Jack McLeod brought his bride to meet Jeannie in Melbourne. He named his daughter Jeannie Gunn McLeod and gave each of his sons the second name Gunn.

Jeannie's flair for picturesque descriptions, heightened by her sense of adventure, made her letters home very entertaining. She faithfully recorded the quaint, picturesque expressions of the bushmen, for example their description of salty damper as "Lot's wife" or an aggressive woman as "a snorter". More importantly, she described their character in a few bold strokes allied to picturesque nicknames. "The Dandy", for example, was named because of a love of orderliness and clean clothing in a land that cared nothing for either, but she hastened to assure her family back home that the man's heart "had not a touch of dandyism in it". The mailman who took these letters was the "Fizzer" because he had to "fizz along" to reach each destination in time, knowing how important mail is to those isolated in the bush. Her family kept all her letters because they enjoyed them so much.

The homestead began to be built in earnest when the itinerant carpenter, Little Johnny, arrived. He always spoke of having "urgent business elsewhere", which he seemed to use to spur himself on. His perpetual cry was, "Now we shan't be long", which cheered them all. Jeannie grew fond of the perky little man who was always on the move. She was saddened, years later, to hear of his untimely death by drowning while crossing a flooded river, striving still to reach that urgent business elsewhere.

With the homestead in better shape, she was at ease entertaining travellers, a surprising number of whom visited, from overlanders to billabongers, owners of stations to stockmen, swagmen and adventurers to government officials. This unending stream appeared from nowhere and disappeared into "sometimes bright memories, sometimes sad, and sometimes little memory at all".

A sense of foreboding, of danger, invaded Jeannie and the little community when one sick traveller died of some unidentified malady. He was buried by his faithful mate next to other unmarked graves on a little rise nearby the homestead. This death posed the unspoken question, "Who will be next in this harsh, unforgiving land?" The answer was to be a little Chinaman who came to them already sick with malarial dysentery. Unfortunately, the wet season always heralded the onset of malaria. Each case was a battle for life in the shadow of death. Some battles were won but others were lost. Jeannie felt helpless each time, lacking medical training and any recourse to a doctor or a supply of medicines. Each episode of illness became a case of making the sick person as comfortable as possible, then waiting.

Finally, personal tragedy struck Jeannie. She closes her account of her thirteen months at Elsey with these words:

> All unaware, that scourge of the Wet crept back to the homestead, and the great Shadow, closing in on us, flung

wide those gates of death once more, and turning before passing through, beckoned to our Maluka [Aeneas] to follow. But at those gates the Maluka lingered a little while with those who were fighting so fiercely and impotently to close them—lingering to teach us out of his own great faith that "Behind all Shadows stands God". And then the gates gently closing, a woman stood alone in that little home.... That is all the world need know. All else lies deep in the silent hearts of the men of the Never-Never—in those great, silent hearts that came to the woman in her need...

Though married for such a short time, Jeannie and Aeneas had shared an especially close bond of love. Jeannie was to form many friendships with a wide variety of men after Aeneas' death, but none of these were romantic relationships. Until her own death sixty years later, Jeannie spoke of Aeneas as "my loving husband".

Immediately after his death, Jeannie moped around the homestead at the Elsey. The Dandy took over the daily responsibilities of management.

Like most relentlessly positive people, Jeannie could none-the-less sink into a black pit of depression and did so. She decided to leave Elsey and never return as every plank, every circumstance, seemed to speak to her of her great loss.

Arrangements were made. Her sister Carrie came to Darwin to meet her and The Dandy accompanied her to the rendezvous. The sisters then sailed to Melbourne where Jeannie was surrounded and comforted by her loving family. Slowly her depression lifted.

Her family and friends had been enthralled by her accounts in her letters of a land and lifestyle about which they knew so little. As time passed, they encouraged her to write a book about her experiences. She could not bring herself to relive her year at Elsey but decided to construct a novel based around Bett-Bett, a young Aboriginal housemaid she had befriended there. She wrote furiously on a low desk in a cane chair using a dip pen and inkpot, which was how pupils worked in the schools of those days. Her home schooling all those years before meant that Jeannie was used to long hours at a desk in her home.

The novel was accepted by publishers but with some adjustments. They changed the title to *The Little Black Princess* and had the author's name changed from "Jeannie Gunn" to "Mrs Aeneas Gunn". It was published in 1905 and drew good reviews, especially for her style. However, while topical, it was rather too fanciful to add a great deal to the understanding of Aboriginal culture. Nevertheless, it was an encouraging start and she decided to tackle next the story of her tumultuous thirteen months at Elsey. Her letters home refreshed her memory and she worked from them.

Jeannie began her account several times, but then put it aside—the memories were simply too bittersweet, too poignant. Finally she determined to complete it as a way of facing and expunging her pain.

We Of The Never-Never was published in 1908 and grew rapidly in popularity and influence, becoming an Australian bush classic that has sold in excess of a million copies. It opened the eyes of the cities to how primitive conditions really were in the outback. But what could be done in a practical way to improve conditions? The fledgling nation had neither the resources nor the resolve to tackle the problems.

One man, though, saw things differently. His name was John Flynn and he was training at Ormond College in Melbourne to become a minister of the Presbyterian Church. In 1909 he experienced a strange but definite call from God to do something about the conditions suffered by the people of the Inland, yet had little idea himself what might be involved. Seeking out information, he was recommended to read *We Of The Never-Never*, which had been published just a few months previously. He was deeply moved by what he read, so much so that he determined to meet the author to discuss what might be attempted in a practical way to help the people of the bush.

Jeannie met Flynn first at her father's house in Creswick Street, Hawthorn. The tall, gangling, bespectacled man in his late twenties and the tiny, sparkling, butterfly that was Jeannie found they had an immediate affinity, perhaps because they were both extraordinarily positive people. Flynn spoke slowly but with well-chosen words and a touch of humour, his blue-grey eyes twinkling behind his round-rimmed spectacles. Her speech was much quicker, but she also injected humour and smiled often to lighten the impact of the sad anecdotes that she told about life in the Territory.

A lifelong friendship was struck that day based around their similar thinking and their mutual concern for the plight of the battlers in the bush. Another thing they found in common was a strong Christian faith.

Their conversation that day gave Flynn much to think about and also heightened his awareness of the potential of literature to minister to the outback, where men were too sparsely spread to visit easily but many of whom loved reading.

Later that same year, he began to plan a little book to help battlers entitled *The Bushman's Companion*. It was a mix of good practical and spiritual advice, nothing very pious, and was finally published in September 1910. It proved an immediate success. He visited Jeannie again to discuss his ideas for a sequel.

"I would like to publish a *Bushwoman's Companion,* full of material that you would have found helpful at Elsey," Flynn told her.

"There are so many things of which I was ignorant before going up North, nearly everything in fact. A book of advice would have been a boon. It's a fine concept."

Together they roughed over some ideas and Jeannie promised to contribute articles to it.

Before Flynn left, she said something that stuck in his mind, "I'm glad that you included a chapter on First Aid in your *Bushman's Companion*. If you are going to help our pioneers in a meaningful way, you will need to take healing to them, for their spirits with the Gospel, but also for their bodies. I went to Elsey a bride and I returned a widow. In the short time I was there three fresh graves were dug in our little cemetery."

Jeannie was to repeat this advice about healing when Flynn went to visit her in 1912 after he had been given his commission to set up a mission to help the pioneers. She added a further dimension of advice that his mission should try to help pioneers socially, because many suffered from loneliness and lack of social interaction. This seemed like an impossible dream when Jeannie voiced the problem because Flynn's pioneers were spread thinly over two million square miles! How could you interact with people you seldom if ever made contact with?

What happened about the *Bushwoman's Companion*? Jeannie contributed articles faithfully, as did others including the pioneer and authoress Jessie Litchfield in the Northern Territory. However, Flynn took an appointment to an itinerant ministry at Beltana in January 1911, an appointment both isolated and demanding. Then after starting his new mission in 1912 he became frantically busy, "My life is not my own any longer," he wrote. The upshot was that the *Bushwoman's Companion* was never published, though a number of the articles Jeannie penned appeared in church magazines like the *Presbyterian Banner* and the *Messenger*.

Meanwhile, life for Jeannie moved on. There was a growing demand from the reading public for more books, so she decided to write something about the bush region in the Dandenong Mountains, near Melbourne. Jeannie loved this area and knew it well as she often went riding there, especially in Sherbrooke Forest. She investigated its history and spoke with the people, and *The Making of Monbulk* began to take shape. She delayed finishing it to go on an overseas tour with her sister and they had a memorable time tripping throughout the British Isles and France. To her surprise, she was given a reception at the Lyceum Club to "honour this brilliant Australian authoress" and was also written up in *La Donna* and other magazines. Modestly, she disclaimed any literary pretensions, "My books are popular because the topics covered are currently of interest," she told the media.

She returned in October 1913 to an Australia gearing up for war and found she could not settle to finish *The Making of Monbulk*, so it was never completed. What she wrote has not survived.

Instead of writing further, Jeannie became distressed by the dislocation of young Australians serving in the Great War. She threw herself wholeheartedly into caring for the young lads who were streaming into the cities to join the army. Many of them were from "up-country" and were naive, needing her motherly help to organise their lives.

Jeannie by now was living with her unmarried sister Elizabeth in Hawthorn. The two were faithful members of Scots Church and always sat together near the front. When hostilities commenced, Jeannie and Elizabeth offered a place through their church for homesick soldiers to have a free meal, home cooking, and a friendly chat. Jeannie gave strict instructions to the maid that the soldiers were to be welcomed and allowed in even if they arrived roaring drunk. She discovered many were confused or worried and welcomed counsel and practical help. The news from the battlefields of Europe was not always good and the youngsters needed encouragement and spiritual guidance also. Once again, Jeannie's wise but gentle nature won her many friendships.

She knitted hundreds of items for the young soldiers, especially warm socks, and took to knitting even as she walked, a ball of wool dangling from a special metal bracelet on her arm. She sent many parcels and wrote hundreds of letters. Her mantelpiece became covered with the photographs sent her by the grateful men. When they returned injured, she helped to solve their problems. When they did not return, she found herself comforting their bereaved families. She, too, knew what it was to lose a loved one cut down before his time.

Jeannie believed that caring for soldiers was what God had dropped into her lap and she was fully occupied doing so. But her literary drive remained too and all the letters she wrote only partially satisfied it.

Over the years she remained in contact with Bett-Bett, the mischievous little Aboriginal girl around whom Jeannie had constructed *The Little Black Princess*. Bett-Bett had left Elsey and found employment in the home of Mrs Ward, who took her to see Jeannie when travelling herself with her family to Melbourne. Bett-Bett begged to stay on in Melbourne with Jeannie, but had shivered with cold during the whole time she was there. Jeannie, wisely, decided Bett-Bett would be happier in the heat of the Territory but wrote to her faithfully throughout her life, keeping the pencil sketch of a kiss and a shell from Bett-Bett on her writing desk always. This continuing friendship made Jeannie wonder whether a serious description of Aboriginal lives and culture might not build a bridge of understanding with other Australians. Therefore, in 1917, she began to prepare *Terrick: His Book*.

Terrick was a tall, courteous Aborigine from the Coranderrk Settlement, close enough that Jeannie could spend time talking with him and observe the habits and customs of the tribe. Because of her involvement helping soldiers, she did not spend as much time with Terrick as she would have liked. When she went, she always took with her squares of blue cloth for the women of Coranderrk as they preferred blue, saying, "It goes with our dark skins". They gave her gifts of basketware in turn. She noted tribal differences from the Aborigines she had known at Elsey and recorded all her observations carefully in notes taken on the spot.

When the war ended, she found herself busier than ever helping the soldiers to resettle. They had multiple problems—personal, emotional and financial. She was a frequent visitor at Caulfield Military Hospital, comforting the sick and crippled. She went often with returning soldiers to the Barracks in St Kilda Road, to ensure they received all of their entitlements, especially as the red tape could prove bewildering to the less-educated fighting man. Over the years, her self-sacrificing service received various commendations, one citation reading appropriately that "she has been one to whom any ex-serviceman could turn in time of trouble". Her selfless efforts on their behalf went on and on for many years, but it was at the expense of her writing.

Then Terrick died. She attended his funeral and also followed the dray to the cemetery where her old friend was interred at twilight as the fog blew up from the Yarra flats. Along with the coffin, into the ground went her desire to try and write his story further. Not even her unfinished notes survive. In fact very little of her writing survives, yet she was in 1939 awarded the OBE for services to Australian literature.

However, one account she completed, though short, had an impact on a young Flying Doctor, Allan Vickers, as he started his career. He was told the story during a visit he and Flynn paid to Jeannie and it deeply affected him. He asked Jeannie to write him out a copy. It appears early on in Vickers' unfinished memoirs. The story concerned Jeannie's "Eastern Neighbour", who was their closest white neighbour to Elsey and who was a courteous, fun-loving and generous friend to them.

As so little of her writing has survived, I will retain Jeannie's account in full although it was not written for publication and does not especially showcase her literary skills.

> Pierce Eaglesfield Smith, of Hodgson Downs cattle station, was our Eastern Neighbour in my book, *We of the Never-Never*. The Hodgson Downs homestead was ninety miles east from the old Elsey Homestead and a little more than that from the Overland Telegraph Line at the present Mataranka.
>
> Sometime during the dry season of 1907, after I had left the Elsey, Mr Smith was out after cattle some forty miles east of his homestead, with a couple of Aborigines in attendance, when his horse put its foot into a rat's burrow and fell, breaking Mr Smith's ankle in its fall and twisting the foot back so badly that the broken ends of both bones of the leg were left protruding right through the skin.
>
> The Aborigines left him where he had fallen, and built a bough "gundi" over him for shelter. Then one of them, at Mr Smith's instructions, rode in the forty miles to the homestead for help, leaving the other in attendance.
>
> The forty-mile ride, without a change of horse, took him well on through the night.
>
> A buckboard was got ready, with relays of horses in the charge of Aborigines to be picked up on the return trip. A stretcher-bed was taken on it, and a white stockman drove out with the Aborigine as guide, taking with him such First Aid as he could contrive.
>
> That journey with all its preparations took until well after the sundown of that second day, and sometime during the third day Mr Smith was carried back into the homestead on the stretcher-bed.
>
> The nearest doctor was in Port Darwin, some 400 miles away and held there by government contract. And so, with the earliest dawn of the fourth day after the accident, there began an appalling drive of 250 miles over the roughest bush tracks and dry creek-beds, to the railhead at Pine Creek. This would be a preliminary to a further 150 miles by train to Port Darwin and treatment.

The buck-board journey took another sixteen or seventeen days; for even though the poor patient was strapped to the wire mattress of his stretcher-bed, if the team went out of a walk, the jolting was unendurable to him. At creek crossings, his stretcher had to be taken out and carried across by hand, and reloaded when the team had been rushed down and across the creek bed. In spite of the utmost care the flies had got to the poor shattered limb, and gradually each day's journey had to be shortened as the patient's strength gave way.

And so, on the seventeenth day from the Hodgson Downs homestead, Pine Creek was sighted. Then, as a last straw, the train chose that exact moment to commence shunting, in preparation for a special express journey to Port Darwin for the patient. The bush horses took fright and bolted, crashing buckboard and patient and all into a tree stump! Freeing themselves, the horses left all there at the roadside.

A nurse had been sent out from the Darwin Hospital to take charge of the case on the train and hurried to the scene. The poor bushman was picked up on his stretcher and boarded onto the waiting train—and travelled express into Darwin.

The leg was amputated below the knee at eleven o'clock that night. It was exactly three weeks after the accident.

Mr Smith, after a five month battle for his life, came South, but died four years later in 1911, never having recovered fully from this terrible happening.

And so the Frontier lost another kind, talented, successful bushman because of the primitive conditions that reigned there.

This account of Jeannie's greatly influenced the kindly Doctor Allan Vickers. Vickers later on became pivotal to the survival and then the development of the Royal Flying Doctor Service. [The RFDS has had a variety of names during its proud history. However, for simplicity, the abbreviation RFDS will be used throughout this book].

Jeannie was especially delighted when Flynn, in 1917, opened an AIM Nursing Home at Maranboy, a mere 50 miles from Elsey station. At last her friends at Elsey and neighbouring stations could obtain help when they fell sick and not have to suffer wretchedly while their helpless loved ones looked on. She knew that her advice to Flynn had contributed towards the development of his nursing homes, and this helped to satisfy her own unfulfilled wish to become a medical missionary. She could not go herself, but others would be there in her place, because of the guidance she had given Flynn. She wrote an enthusiastic letter to him that he treasured amongst his personal possessions and was on his desk when he died:

> This is the best—perhaps the only—true advance the poor old Territory has made in the last five or six years. What a hospital and nurse will mean out there only those who have known utter helplessness when a beloved life is at stake can ever quite realise.

What of her other friends from Elsey days?

The Fizzer, Henry Peckham, was their mailman who braved a rugged circuit of 1600 kilometres to bring them mail eight times a year. Henry worried about the dry stretches, always aware that his predecessor had perished of thirst in one of them. Despite his gruelling route, he was so punctual that it was said you could set your clock by him. This passion for getting the mail through on time proved to be his undoing, but ironically from flood and not thirst. In April 1911 he found the Victoria River raging and blocking his path, so he put his horse in to test the current and was swept away and drowned. His last words, shouted back to his Aboriginal assistant, were, "Don't put the packs [of mail] in, it's too strong!" His body was found later and buried beside the river.

The Dandy, H.H. Bryant, finally left the Territory in 1918 and married in Angaston, South Australia. He and Jeannie met from time to time. Jeannie was extremely fond of his baby daughter, whom she dubbed "The Wee Dandy". He and the Quiet Stockman, Jack McLeod, lie buried in the same graveyard in Angaston.

Cheon, the cook, spoke often of his time at the Elsey. Then, in 1919, Jeannie received this message by telegram from Darwin:

GOODBYE MISSIE STOP ME GO LONGA CHINA

Jeannie did not expect to hear from Cheon again, but in 1922 received a letter. He sent her a beautiful blue silk embroidered tablecloth and his best wishes for health and great happiness, but mentioned that he meanwhile was feeble and could hardly walk anymore. It was his farewell.

Bett-Bett married and became Mrs Bonson and lived near Darwin. She was described years later as "a very sweet old lady" and was the only one of Jeannie's friends at Elsey to outlive the author.

Shortly before his death, when asked about possible memorials in his honour, the great John Flynn had quietly demurred. When pressed, he surprised everyone by saying that if a monument were to be erected he would prefer it at the old Elsey homestead. His statement appears to have been disregarded, perhaps thought to be an expression of humility. But some AIM nurses heard of it through Sister Grace Francis and comprehended what was really in Flynn's heart, that he wanted to honour the brave "Little Missus" who had struggled against impossible odds at Elsey and whose life and advice had been so inspiring to him. Flynn's nurses quietly set about raising the necessary money themselves.

On the seventh anniversary of Flynn's death, the AIM Nursing Sisters placed a cairn and brass plaque at the old Elsey homestead just as he had wanted. It commemorates Jeannie Gunn's book and marks the site of the old homestead, now destroyed by fire and the attentions of souvenir hunters. However, one part of that era has survived rather better, the Elsey Cemetery. During the Second World War soldiers worked hard to establish it, partly in recognition of Jeannie's outstanding commitment to their wellbeing over many years. Aeneas is buried there. His confident words to Jeannie just before his death are quoted boldly on his tombstone,

BEHIND ALL SHADOWS STANDETH GOD

Jeannie never saw that tombstone apart from in a photograph. She said when she left the Elsey that she would never return and that was how she lived, true to every statement she made.

Jeannie enjoyed a lavish ninetieth birthday celebration in 1960. She was chirpy, positive and full of fun and remained so throughout her final year of life. She died on 9th June 1961, aged 91 years, happy and surrounded by many friends. It had been nearly six decades earlier that she had travelled out to the Elsey as a bride and into her place in pioneering folklore.

Jeannie gave Flynn a comprehensive understanding of what life had been like for her in the Territory at the turn of the century. Her penetrating insights helped to guide him throughout his life.

Flynn had a wide circle of friends and acquaintances who informed him of the problems in parts of Australia other than the Territory. In the next chapter we read what some of them told him.

2

SNIPPETS ABOUT PIONEERING WOMEN AND THE CONDITIONS THEY FACED

Thousands of pages have been written about the rugged lifestyles of pioneer women. I will limit myself to four accounts, each by a friend of Flynn's or by a colleague of his visionary endeavours.

We begin with Hudson Fysh, who was a co-founder of Qantas Airlines and a good friend and advisor of Flynn's. He wrote a book, *Taming the North,* about the old pioneer Andrew Kennedy, who was one of the original Directors of Qantas and actually its first paying passenger on an air route. Kennedy invested heavily in Qantas and influenced young Fysh into supporting the Flying Doctor concept. The reasons for his enthusiasm for Flynn's vision are to be found in the hardships he and his family suffered.

Here is an incident taken from *Taming the North*. Kennedy and his family, along with his wife's sister Mrs Currie and her own family, sold their property in Northern Queensland in 1881 and set out to settle elsewhere:

> The party, consisting of Mr and Mrs Kennedy and their three children and Mr and Mrs Currie and their three, set out in high hopes for Cloncurry. The means of conveyance were horses for the men, and a spring-cart and horse-dray for the women and children and their belongings. The elder children rode in turns.
>
> It was a very wet year, the monsoonal rains breaking early and descending in a deluge such as is seen only in the tropics. The usually hard bush track became a bog of impeding mud where the black-soil flats were crossed, clinging to the floundering feet of the horses and clogging the wheels of the vehicles. The party struggled on till Rocky Waterhole near Chatsworth was reached; at which point the swollen waters formed a bar to further progress. Ahead were more creeks, also impassable, and there was nothing for it but to camp and await a cessation of the rain and a

subsidence of the rushing torrents of water that overflowed the creek-beds.

Tents were pitched and all made themselves as comfortable as possible under the circumstances; but the rain continued day after day with no sign of ceasing.

The delay became agonising for there was another reason for haste. Mrs Currie was expecting a child at any time! It had been hoped to reach Cloncurry before the event took place.

Still the creeks remained up and over a week went by.

Mrs Currie's child was born in a tent by the roadside with the rain still beating down and the roaring creek in front.

Under these conditions, it is no wonder that several days afterwards, Mrs Currie was taken seriously ill with dysentery. The infant son also became ill, as did her second youngest child, a boy. Norman, Mrs Kennedy's youngest child, also fell sick.

A fight for their lives followed, but it was an unequal contest owing to the damp and unsuitable conditions and the absence of proper nourishment and medicines.

Mrs Currie and her two sons passed away, but Norman was saved. He owed his life to a pony that had been brought with them. Having just had a young foal, it provided milk that the youngster was able to take.

A grave was dug by the roadside and into it were lowered the bodies of Mrs Currie and her two little sons. Kennedy read the burial service and then erected a strong log fence round the grave where sleep this pioneer woman and her two children. The rude posts that mark the place have long since rotted away.

Mrs Kennedy loved her sister, and the long companionship in circumstances of bravery and hardship so rudely broken left an impression that, after the passage of fifty years, she could look back only with the deepest sadness and feeling.

Today in carrying out his errand of mercy to far-off Boulia and Birdsville, the Flying Doctor *wings his way over that very spot*, soaring over flood and plain, doing in a few hours what it took the pioneers weeks to accomplish. It was a great source of satisfaction to Kennedy in later life that the Aerial

Medical Service Headquarters, one of the first such pioneering services in the world, and the first in Australia, was established at his home town of Cloncurry; and that he took a hand in the inauguration of this wonderful boon to the outback, through the agency of Qantas, who are identified with the flying side of the organization.

It would no doubt have been a matter of further pride for Andrew Kennedy had he known his granddaughter, Sister Heather Kennedy, would one day serve in Flynn's network of safety. She went to the cottage hospital at Fitzroy Crossing in 1953.

* * * *

Flynn had many letters cross his desk written by women who portrayed the difficulties of their lives in the bush. Here are excerpts from one he quoted in the October 1918 *Inlander*:

> To the nearest post office is ninety miles one way, and then there is another small township 116 miles the other way. We have to trust to the boundary rider on the Border Fence to carry our mail, what little there is, as we have no government mail close out here.
>
> My nearest neighbour is seventeen miles away, but just at present they are forty miles away: they had to shift, no feed for the stock. We are having a very bad time here this last twelve months, and rain is wanted badly.
>
> It is sometimes twelve months before I see another woman, but I don't seem to mind a bit now I have got quite used to it. At first it was terrible. I only had one little baby and my husband would be away for ten or twelve days at a time. I now have three children.

Letters like these made Flynn very determined to establish wireless communications in the Inland so that women could at least talk to neighbours, even if they could seldom meet face to face. "The dumb bush must learn to speak," he proclaimed. "It is not fair that our brave pioneers should struggle on alone without friendship, nor have any avenue to get advice in times of crisis".

* * * *

Flynn knew firsthand the fear of sickness in extremes of isolation. Besides combating loneliness, the concept of wireless communications and Flying Doctors was designed to lessen that nagging fear. Edith Miller describes what it was like to carry the responsibility for medical treatment for her family and others on an isolated cattle station in Western Australia:

> I first went North as a young bride, in 1923. It was a stark place to live. We had no electricity, gas, telephone, car, freezer or wireless. We had a staff of 12 permanent men, a few casuals and a hundred Aboriginals living in the camp on our property. Caring for everyone's health fell upon my narrow shoulders. When bad colds swept the Aboriginal camp, there would be a sick parade at the store each morning after breakfast and a spoonful of medicine poured into each open mouth in the line. It had to be a very severe case, beyond my scope, to tackle the rough bush roads into Port Hedland.
>
> One of the most agonising times was when our small daughter of two-and-a-half years was very ill with enteritis. Unusual rains had made the roads to the doctor 180 miles away impassable, and there was another baby on the way. So my husband sent an Aborigine cross-country on a horse to the small mining town of Bamboo Creek, with a note for the storekeeper to read to the matron at Marble Bar on the phone. She located a truck leaving that very day in our direction and gave the driver the medicine that would help. He drove through the night to bring us what proved to be the turning point for a very sick little girl and heartfelt relief to two worried parents.
>
> And again, I remember a time when Johnny, a young black of perhaps 10 or 11 years old, had slipped and fallen on some sheets of corrugated iron and cut the calf of his left leg, leaving a great lump of flesh hanging.
>
> Something had to be done immediately. My husband sterilised a spool of white linen thread and some saddler's needles, and swabbing the area with antiseptic, stitched it up. The gallant little boy never uttered a sound. As for me, I went away and lost all the food I had eaten that day.

No wonder the Millers asked for, and got, the first Flying Doctor transceiver in Western Australia on their cattle station, Warrawagine. And during the ceremony to inaugurate the first Flying Doctor Base in Western Australia, Dr Allan Vickers received an emergency call from Edith. Dramatically, he left the ceremony at once and flew out to their property to rescue an Aborigine with spinal injuries.

Relief from the responsibility for serious medical cases had at last come for Edith. She wrote to Flynn expressing her gratitude.

Edith wanted to do something tangible to help Flynn's work. Later on she spent many years as a speaker and fund-raiser for the RFDS and in 1969 was awarded the MBE in recognition of her outstanding efforts.

* * * *

Our fourth writer was a pioneering woman herself and had great insight into the true situation faced by women in the bush. In this account she scorns an Englishwoman whose pretentious intention it was to "civilise those crude women" who inhabited the Australian bush:

> We received an object lesson on how NOT to live in the north Australian bush when a gentleman, recently arrived from "Home" [England], took up a selection on the Daly River, and decided to have his wife out there with him. She also was a new arrival, London-born and bred, without the slightest knowledge of bush life. She brought all her furniture with her to Darwin, for transhipment to the Daly. Darwin folk, although admiring her piano, silver cake-baskets, brocade-covered chairs, bevelled-glass mirrors, aluminium cooking utensils, egg-shell china, and silver cutlery, warned her that such furniture would be a burden to her in the bush, and they advised her to store all her costly goods in Darwin, just to take the plainest and simplest things with her to the Daly. Unfortunately, she did not follow this advice; possibly in imagination she saw herself as a pioneer of civilization in the bush, setting the outback women an example.

All her elaborate furniture was sent up to the Daly by lugger, much to its skipper's disgust; for the bulkier articles had to be stowed on deck, where they were soon stained with sea-spray and eaten by cockroaches.

When they arrived at the Daly, all the furniture had to be temporarily stowed under tarpaulins; for Mrs Englishwoman discovered that the "commodious Colonial mansion" she had imagined was simply a bark humpy, some ten feet by twelve, with an ant-bed floor. Borers ate her elaborate furniture; white ants destroyed her sideboards; ginger ants built in her piano, and cockroaches lived in her brocaded chairs. Frogs, centipedes and spiders made uninvited calls upon her; open fires blackened her aluminium cooking-utensils, soon bumped out of shape by the clumsy fingers of the blacks, who also stole all her silver cutlery.

When the Wet set in, lace curtains, embroidered bedspreads, and toilet covers became mildewed in a single night; her crocodile dressing-case grew hoary whiskers, and the glued portions became unstuck; her elaborate house-gowns, tea-gowns and rest-gowns became discoloured with wet bark, blackened with mildew, and eaten into holes by cockroaches and crickets. Her husband's evening dress suits made a meal for the white ants along with the camphor-wood chest that housed them.

So a very unhappy English couple abandoned their selection in disgust, and returned to their London flat, leaving the bush-women still unconverted.

Jessie Litchfield wrote the above in her book, *Far North Memories*, published in 1930. Contrast this Englishwoman's attitude with Jessie's own positive and practical approach to living in the bush, described by her in these words:

> Out bush, you simply had to be able to turn your hand to anything. I soled my own shoes; mended leaks in frying pans and saucepans by soldering with iron and flux; helped my husband build the humpy we lived in; made my own bread, lemon butter, potted meat and chilli drinks; made ginger beer; went prospecting with my husband if he wanted to test a likely spot; taught my children by correspondence; and constructed most of my own

furniture. The blacks used to bring us bags full of kapok, which grew wild in the bush, and I made my own mattresses and pillows and cushions, which lasted for years.

She also produced all the family's clothes, shoes, hats, curtains, tablecloths, sheets and mattress covers—and she used to bake 18 loaves of bread every day!

Jessie's resourcefulness and hard work were typical of pioneering women of that era, but in other ways her life was most unusual. She was a pivotal influence on Flynn and wrote the letter in 1909 that turned his life around.

Her biography begins on the next page.

3

The Inspiration—Jessie Litchfield

While training to be a Minister in the Presbyterian Church, John Flynn volunteered to become a missionary to Korea. Extraordinarily talented, he may well have become "Flynn of Korea" instead of "Flynn of the Inland" had this letter not come across his path:

> West Arm, Port Darwin, 3/6/1909.
>
> Dear Mrs Kelly,
> I expect you will be surprised at this letter from a total stranger, but I was, before my marriage, a member of the Richmond Presbyterian Church. I received some copies of its monthly paper, and I am writing now some news of this lonely land.
> I am eighty miles from a town by land, twenty miles by sea, three miles from the nearest white woman, two miles from the nearest white man. Chinese and blacks are my nearest neighbours -there is a Catholic priest, a Church of England clergyman, and lay preachers at the Methodist Church (all in Darwin vicinity)—there are no other ministers in the Northern Territory—500,000 square miles [1.3 million sq. km] of country with 1500 whites, 2000 Chinese and 5000 blacks living there.
> Of the whites, fully 500 of the men keep lubras [black women] or use them as they want them, and nearly all have half-caste illegitimate children whose only future in life is prostitution. There are not 50 Chinese without lubras. There is no law against this evil, and there are no missionaries to teach the people right from wrong - I know that drink, drugs and lubras are responsible for nine out of ten hospital cases, and also for seven deaths out of ten.
> Why cannot the Presbyterian Church send up a missionary to the Northern Territory; an earnest, enthusiastic married man (he is better married than single),

give him one hundred pounds for living expenses, a certain sum for travelling expenses, and let him make his headquarters in Darwin and have regular periods for visiting the outer places of the NT? He would do good if he were a man who put Christ first, and who worked for the good of others, and spared neither time nor money nor labour in the cause of Christ.

You may be shocked by this letter, but I have understated rather than overstated the facts.

Yours faithfully,
Jessie Litchfield.

Flynn recorded later that something stirred deep within him as he read this letter and that he was not able to get it off his mind. Before reading it, he had not visualised the vast Australian Inland as a potential mission field. But within days he decided God was calling him to become a missionary to outback Australia and not to Korea at all. So he resigned from the Korean mission and focused his attention on the vast parched Inland instead.

Flynn carried Jessie's letter around with him everywhere. He got together a group of women in Melbourne that included his sister Rosetta and her friend, Esther Mahood, and showed it to them. One of the women there that day described its impact in the *Victorian Messenger*:

> It was a letter that left you crying out, almost in hatred, against the writer for daring to show you such ugly things, for the knowledge of them robbed you of something... But that is small I suppose, and weak, though desperately womanlike and we had need to rise above it.

Stirred by compassion, these women began to support Flynn's initiatives to help the pioneers. They formed the Mailbag League, which sent letters and packages of books and other items to isolated and deprived folk in the bush. Flynn also garnered his sister, who wrote the "Cousin Charlotte" column in the *Messenger*, and the devout Esther Mahood, to start a drive to raise awareness of the plight of the pioneers. Esther would write in letters of protest regarding the conditions in the bush that Cousin Charlotte published. Flynn sent Esther a pile of letters collected from his patrol area near Oodnadatta for her to quote from. In this way Rosetta and Esther raised funds that enabled Flynn to undertake a survey of conditions in the Northern Territory and the outback in general. Excited at the prospect, he wrote to Jessie Litchfield, who had penned the letter that had turned his life around, and arranged to meet her in Darwin. What type of young woman would he meet there?

Indeed, who was the woman that had written so influential a letter in 1909 at the comparatively young age of twenty-six? And what was she doing in the rough and earthy North?

* * * *

Jessie Litchfield had exceptional talent even in childhood. Dame Mary Gilmore, who is recognised as one of Australia's leading women of letters, wrote of her, "When I first met Jessie Litchfield [then Jessie Phillips] she was about twelve and a pupil in my class at Neutral Bay, Sydney Public School. Even then she stood out in character, personality and intelligence. All that life had to do was develop her."

How, then, did life develop this child with so much promise?

She enjoyed a happy childhood, involved in her school, church and family activities. A vibrant and sociable teenager, she had a number of young men interested in her, but she entered her twenties without having formed any serious romantic relationships.

Then her world fell apart. Her beloved parents separated. Her sensitive soul felt betrayed and she expressed this in poetry:

> PARTING
> 'Tis hard to hear the unkind tones
> That cause the tears to start,
> But from the friends we dearly love
> 'Tis harder still to part.

A disillusioned Jessie was sent by her family to relatives in China in 1907, quite soon after the family unit had finally torn apart. It was thought the holiday would help her to recover her good spirits. It certainly did that, but long before the ship reached

China, because she had a whirlwind shipboard romance with a young engineer and miner named Valentine Litchfield. He was tall and handsome, with curly hair and bright eyes and a friendly, charming manner. Within three days he had persuaded her to marry him and when he disembarked in Darwin was most reluctant to allow her to continue to China. He was insecure about her returning to him. She, however, still needed time and space away from Australia to combat the conflicts within her.

Six months later Jessie returned to Port Darwin. She intended to spend three weeks there to discover whether her earlier romance with Valentine might develop further.

Once again, the charming miner whirled her off her feet and she soon postponed her return to the South and anything that remained there for her.

Jessie had been an enthusiastic member of the Presbyterian Church in Richmond, Melbourne, with which Flynn was associated. She had found friendship and a personal faith in God there and was determined to have a church wedding. She met the minister of Darwin's Knuckey Street Methodist church and arranged to be married there on 21st of January 1908. Valentine was twenty-three and she a year older.

The young bride needed both her faith and her love of Val to sustain her when they crossed by launch to West Arm. They had to walk eight hot kilometres along a rough track through rainforest to their home. Val organised and paid Aborigines to carry their luggage. But Jessie ignored the difficulties and, with her poet's eye for beauty, found their walk "an enchanting road through a fairyland of delight", loving the multicoloured leaves and bright bird life that flitted past. To her, in her vigorous youth, this was a pathway to a new paradise with the man she loved so very much.

"I warned you it would be a bit rough," Val said in his easygoing, nonchalant way when they eventually arrived at the "house" in which they would start their married life.

That was an understatement. It was no more than a shack with hessian sacking for walls and an iron roof that would turn it into an oven during the heat of the day. There were no windows, but there was ample ventilation and light because a gap had been left between walls and roof and walls and floor. A bough shed made exclusively of timber and leaves in front of it was designed to provide shade during the very hot hours.

Jessie went inside. "A beer-case did duty as a dressing table and a cement cask served the purpose of a washstand. The kitchen held the stove, the water-barrel and a long bench, which did duty both as wash-up bench and cooking table. The sitting room boasted a table with legs fixed into the floor, several stools contrived from meat cases, two or three home-made deck-chairs covered with kangaroo skins, and a small hanging safe which protected sugar, milk etc. from intrusive ants... Although so scantily furnished, the place was neat and home like. A few favourite authors reposed on a small shelf above the household supplies and a few pictures, carefully chosen from illustrated newspapers, decorated the walls."

Val watched Jessie carefully as she inspected the home. "No matter that it is rough," she concluded. "We will soon get it ship-shape." He was relieved at her cheerful response. He had married a "good un", all right!

A home of her own! For the first few days Jessie worked hard to improve it. She found that there were advantages to having few worldly goods because it meant less cleaning, and the ant-bed floors needed only a daily damping and sweeping to be kept in perfect order. Rubbish that would not burn was buried; therefore there was no unsightly litter lying about the house—and empty tins and broken bottles were not left lying about the camp to catch water and breed mosquitoes.

Her main challenge was to adjust her life to fit in with Val's shift work on the drills. For example, when his shift began at midnight he would turn in to sleep at sundown and she would wait up, reading or sewing, to prepare him his supper before he set out and would also make sure he had a steaming breakfast waiting when he came home dirty and tired the next morning. Food preparation was not as easy as in the cities, as it all had to be done from scratch, but they did not lack variety:

> We sampled many kinds of food at West Arm. Fresh beef was almost unprocurable, though now and again a Chinaman would drive a small bullock across from a nearby station, when it would be killed, cut up, and sold around the different mining camps. But bush birds were plentiful; we used their bodies to make soups or pies, and their eggs were delicious in puddings and custards. Quail were in millions on the flats, and quail-on-toast, with fried mushrooms that grew on the sandy flats and the tailing heaps, although very small, were deliciously sweet. Those same tailing heaps, great mounds of sand and mica, grew most wonderful melons and pumpkins in the wet season—great lumps of sweetness that literally melted in the mouth. We usually adjourned to the tailing heaps in the evenings, scooping out seats in the soft sand, and resting there.

She and Valentine shared a love of nature and took long walks. They chatted with the various men they met along the path, there being around eighty white miners and a hundred Chinese in the area. They also swam in the sparkling waters of the tidal creeks or read voraciously any newspapers or magazines that came their way.

Her happiness and energy leapt out of everything she wrote about her life at West Arm, it was indeed her "paradise". And her observations of life there were typically penetrating:

> There were two Chinese storekeepers on the Arm, and, as usual in such out-of-the-way places, they both ran sly-grog shops. But although the drinking may have been heavy occasionally, the stores were conducted decently and respectably; no cause for local criticism ever arose. There was a fair amount of opium smuggling, the Chinese usually proving more than a match for the local police. It was suspected that the occasional small hauls of opium pounced on by the police, "from information received", were designedly planted so that a big batch could be smuggled through in comfort—a sprat to catch a mackerel idea.

The young bride began to long for the company of other women, the closest being Mrs Norman Bell, who lived 12 kilometres away and with whom she formed a life-long friendship. Jessie began spending one day a week with her, walking over in the cool of the morning and returning in the evening. Another long walk she took was to collect the mail from the launch every three weeks.

Jessie wrote the influential letter that inspired Flynn while she was at West Arm. The friendly letter that John Flynn wrote in reply caught Jessie quite by surprise. However, she was delighted that someone might be taking an interest in the dreadful social conditions that prevailed in the Northern Territory. They began a correspondence which led to their eventually meeting in Darwin in 1912, but a lot of water was to pass under the bridge before then in both their lives.

Fever struck the miners at West Arm in 1910. Jessie and Mrs Bell did the best they could in difficult circumstances to tend to the sick men. Fortunately, the malaria was "benign" and deaths did not occur. The problems they faced gave Jessie first hand experience with which to brief Flynn by letter.

Jessie's "paradise time" at West Arm came to an end abruptly after two happy years. The drill cores showed there was insufficient mineral wealth under the surface for the mining company to maintain its interests and without much warning they were told to pack up and get ready to move on. Where to? Remote Anson Bay, 240 kilometres from Darwin. It was the worst possible time for the Litchfields to move somewhere so remote as Jessie was heavily pregnant.

She gave birth to her first baby, Valentine Sinclair Litchfield, just before husband Val was due to sail to Anson Bay. They were both thrilled. Jessie penned a poem to express her wonder and delight. In it we see expressions of her inner character, firstly of her faith and then of her conviction that parents carry an awesome responsibility for how their child turns out.

Valentine Sinclair

The headline written. Nothing more we know.
The scroll unfolds a leaf of virgin white;
And as we gaze upon its spotless snow
Our hearts o'erbrim with wonder and delight

> Yet trembling mingles with the joy and praise;
> A terror lest our hands, despite our care,
> Should mar the spotless page on which we gaze
> Or leave a print of careless fingers there.
>
> Until the Father who bestowed the scroll
> Receives it back into his hands again
> No mark may be erased from off the roll;
> What e're we write, forever must remain.
>
> Therefore we pray, that, as the leaves unfold,
> We write all truth, all purity, and love;
> Until it shines, illumined with purest gold,
> Fit treasure for the Father's house above.

Baby Valentine was just six weeks old when Jessie climbed aboard a pearling lugger to Anson Bay. It was a hot, unpleasant voyage.

Three days later the lugger ran up onto a sandbank and the captain told Jessie she would have to wade ashore from there, a good kilometre and a half through water known to harbour crocodiles and sharks, but there was no alternative on offer. So, clutching her precious bundle tightly, Jessie prepared herself for the challenge:

> Dropping over the side of the lugger into water reaching to our knees, we started off bravely. There were several sandbanks between the lugger and the shore, which was quite a mile away, but we could distinguish a number of bark humpies near the beach. In the gullies between the sand banks the tide ran swiftly, and the water was nearly waist-deep, but we waded along cheerfully, although I tried very hard not to think too often of sharks and alligators [sic].

The "bark humpies" she had seen from the lugger did not belong to Aborigines, as she had supposed, but were the crude camp of the diamond drillers and her new home.

Resourceful and willing as ever, Jessie set about making her new home comfortable. It was certainly unusual and very rugged—the floor was of white seashells and two huge Eugenia apple trees that grew from inside the house held up the bark roof.

"Here, I've got a present for you," Val told her laconically and handed over a large revolver. "It is an eight-chambered German model and I have a thousand cartridges to fit it. I also have a sporting rifle with five hundred cartridges." He laughed at her obvious bewilderment as she gingerly accepted the weapon. "I will show you how to use it," he promised. "I don't know whether you remember hearing about the Bradshaw murders? They took place not too far from here and so I want you to be careful. Now don't panic. The Aborigines aren't hostile, just wilder than those we knew at West Arm. We don't anticipate problems but need to be vigilant. There are only fourteen whites and more than six hundred of them."

Jessie rapidly became a good shot. She slept at night with the revolver under her pillow, fully loaded. As a precaution, she never left the house without strapping the revolver to her belt where it was very visible. All the men also walked around fully armed, just in case, and in pairs around corroboree-time when the Aborigines became very excited and their numbers swelled alarmingly. Jessie wrote graphically of one such "making-young-man" celebration:

> At least one thousand blacks must have taken part in the dancing and singing. The thud, thud, of dancing feet, and the clap, slap, of hands on thighs, and the throbbing of a dozen or so didgeridoos, made sleep impossible. We therefore spent the night strolling up and down the beach, watching the various performers. Of course we were well armed, keeping our revolvers exposed, although had that horde of myalls [bush Aboriginal men] so desired they could have swept us all out of existence in a moment. However, we had invariably treated the blacks with kindness, neither spoiling them with over-indulgence, nor cowing them with cruelty; hence we had little to fear.

She was the only woman at Anson Bay for the first nine months, but surprisingly this made her feel more secure. She explains: "I never needed to use the gun because my baby and myself were adored by the blacks."

Years later Jessie became an enthusiastic member of the Darwin Rifle Club.

Correspondence between Jessie and John Flynn took on another focus. Flynn solicited articles from her for his planned *Bushwoman's Companion*. He became too busy and never published it, but some of Jessie's advice, including bush recipes and how to use an anthill as an oven, found their way into the *Messenger* and other church newspapers.

Forever curious, Jessie was fascinated by the Aborigines at Anson Bay and spent a great deal of time talking with them and studying them. By and large, her observations were sympathetic and favourable:

> I saw a number of corroborees, such as the snake corroboree, the "making young man" corroboree, spear-dances, and special ceremonies for special occasions, such as rain-making and the like. We were always the invited guests at these functions, for we would never have dreamed of "gate-crashing"; it would be the worst of bad manners and the end of all friendships with the Aboriginals, who are the politest of people. It is only the civilised man who can afford to be rude and ill mannered.
>
> The coastal blacks were of a very fine type, tall upstanding men who walked like kings of the earth, who lived on the best of food, and who had the sea and the billabongs to bathe in. They were always in the pink of condition. [Obesity came later with the introduction of refined European foods, notably sugar and white flour, to the diet.]
>
> Unprincipled white men outrage the blackfellows' wives or daughters, yet, when the black tracks down and kills the ravisher, a war of extermination starts. Fully nine out of every ten murders in the North have been due, directly or in part, to unauthorised interference with gins [black women]. Not all the true facts ever get into print, of course, but those who have been privileged to look behind the scenes know more than the general public can ever know, or will ever want to know.
>
> Yes, we may despise our natives; some may think them better off the earth and feel no grief at the thought of their extinction. Yet they feel joy and sorrow, pain and pleasure as we do. A black mother can joyfully welcome her first-born,

and, losing him, grieve for more than half a lifetime. Death can kill her baby; it is powerless against her love... Inferiority is a matter of environment. That old lubra [black woman] would be a ghastly failure in a drawing room, but she could exist in one. On the other hand her white sister transported to the bush would perish miserably.

Jessie was sympathetic to Aborigines at all times and wrote articles of support to newspapers over the years. But she was also realistic regarding some of their traditions that were barbaric and she was just as direct and honest in describing these. At no time was she "politically correct"; rather she told things as she found them. A dramatic example was when the old lubras told her about the feasts they had enjoyed of human flesh. A little prodding disclosed that unwanted babies were especially desirable. In fact, mixed-race babies met this fate most often because "him no more white fella, him no more black fella, him just nussing: him half-caste".

Jessie was shocked further to discover the Aborigines were waiting expectantly for a certain birth to occur in their camp because they wanted to feast on the mixed-race baby.

"It's awful, what can we do?" she asked Valentine.

"We won't let it happen," he replied simply.

"But what if we are moved on again, before the birth?"

They weren't. And the baby was born, and was soon cherished as much as any other baby in the camp. His pureblood Aboriginal half-brother became his best friend.

It is important to note that Jessie never actually saw cannibalism and all her reports were hearsay. However, she gathered a great deal of secondary information that influenced her thinking. Her keen observations were written to different newspapers and magazines at the time and over the years, as her knowledge grew. Since then they have been quoted as authoritative by serious researchers such as Ellen Kettle in her *Health Services in the Northern Territory—a History*. Taking excerpts:

> Jessie Litchfield, living near Delissaville about 1908, had good reason to expect to see many mixed race infants but obviously pregnant women would later deny they had delivered an infant.—p. 42

> Jessie Litchfield, living at an oil drilling camp at the mouth of the Daly River, discussed the fate of mixed-race infants. If the father acknowledged the baby then it was recognised as a person and was reared, but those not owned by their fathers were disposed of at birth.—p. 21
>
> That unwanted infants were cooked and eaten is possibly correct as comments to this effect were made by responsible people—Inspector Foelsche, Mr WG Stretton at Borroloola and Mrs JS Litchfield at Delissaville. Much later, in the 1930s, Mr HE Thonemann at Elsey Cattle station offered extra food rations for women who would keep and rear their infants. Noting the paucity of children in the Aboriginal camp, Mr Thonemann asked the women about this and they admitted quite openly that they were killing them at birth, mostly by pinching their nostrils.—p. 41

Jessie did not blame the Aborigines for their tribal practices but her attitude to certain pioneers was different. She kept her sharpest censure for those white men who not only knew what was happening but also sometimes encouraged it. A certain white man at Daly River came in for special censure because between eight to ten of his progeny had been disposed of based on his advice that "No good you keep em half-caste".

To gain further insight into Jessie's thinking, I quote here from her book, *Far North Memories*, published in 1930. On page 59 we read:

> So far as I could find out by judicious questioning, cannibalism is restricted to the eating of half-castes and other unwanted babies, and to enemies captured by the tribe. It is mainly psychical in inception, for the enemies, women included, are said to bestow their best characteristics on their eaters. Unwanted babies bring good luck to those who feed on them. There are white men living in the North today who are known to have encouraged, or at the least ignored, the eating of their own unwanted half-caste children, even up to the number of nine or ten babies. The blacks see nothing immoral in these feasts, which have been held from time immemorial; but of course such orgies do not take place near towns, but out-back rather.

Based on what she had learned, Jessie later recommended the removal of mixed-race babies and young children from Aboriginal camps during the important 1923 Committee of Inquiry held in Darwin. The opinions expressed at that inquiry, hers included, helped to formulate future policy in regard to children of mixed race. With hindsight and recent revelations regarding the "Stolen Generation" we may disagree with her advice, but it would be hard to disagree with the logic and Christian compassion whence it came.

At Anson Bay, the drill crew lived in close proximity for protection and life was very sociable. "We had brought several packs of cards down to Anson Bay with us, and we played almost every night. Poker was first favourite but nap, crib, euchre and whist all had their turn. Our stakes were strictly limited to matches, but the fun was always fast and furious. Sometimes we held impromptu concerts when stories, recitations, songs and phonograph selections made the evening pass very pleasantly. The blacks were greatly taken by the phonograph and they never tired of listening to it. As soon as the music began, fire-sticks could be seen bobbing along through the jungle in every direction; and soon there would be a mob of blacks gathering round near the house listening in absolute silence until the last note had died away."

Dreaded malaria struck the camp and Jessie and the others fought it stoically. Despite high fevers, no one died. However, it did leave an evil deposit lurking in at least one man's brain.

Jessie discovered she was pregnant in the middle of 1911. She decided to return to her mother and other family members in the South to have the baby. How well would they relate to one another after nearly five years? Her experiences had changed her greatly, and they would have changed too. Jessie had grown "more matronly with the passing years, and her face was browned by the Territory sun and wind, but her eyes were still very clear and her voice was as happy as ever".

Their second child, Boyne, was born in Melbourne in the February of 1912.

Jessie was surprised how much she missed the Territory and, of course, Val. "I soon tired of town life. People were kind to me, but we were out of touch with each other. I felt shut-in in an ordinary bedroom; I longed to feel the night winds stirring my hair. Then I learned to hate the dull, dirty streets; the young fellows hanging about smoking and spitting seemed much more ill-bred and common than the naked myalls I had met in the bush." Typically, she expressed herself in verse:

CITY AND BUSH

How crowded the city,
How grimy the street;
How dreary and gritty
The heart of the city
Whenever we meet.
How crowded the city;
How grimy the city.

The bushland is calling
How can I delay?
Quick cloud-shadows falling
And bush voices calling
Entreating, enthralling—
So how can I stay?
The bushland is calling,
How can I delay?

Nor did she delay. She brought the day of her departure forward. "And so three months had barely passed before I was again on the *Empire*, en route for Darwin, and whispering fervently to myself as the vessel drew away from the wharf, 'Never again!'"

Her emancipation from her roots in the southern cities was now complete. From that time forward, she would be an ardent Territorian and her energies would be spent trying to further its cause alone.

Not long after her return to Anson Bay, the diamond drillers were told to evacuate to Yam Creek.

That same year, 1912, John Flynn met Jessie during his "survey" visit to the North. They had long and fruitful discussions. When he returned South, having spoken with many people, he produced the report that was presented to the General Assembly in September and from which the AIM grew.

For Val and Jessie, there followed a bewildering series of moves to new and unusual locations. Jessie described this adventurous life in her unpublished *Out With The Diamond Drillers*. But it all ended at Pine Creek when the results from the drill cores were so poor that drilling ceased and the men had to look elsewhere for work.

What should they do? They were both in their thirties and had five children. Their way of life had been wonderful but had not really fitted them for much else. Their situation would be difficult enough today, but was perilous before the era of social welfare had been established. Fortunately, Val found work on a mine at Union Reefs, about sixteen kilometres from Pine Creek. Jessie and kids lived in a bark humpy three kilometres out of town and it was a lonely life after the comradeship of the diamond drillers. With time on her hands, though, Jessie wrote many articles for southern and local newspapers. This effort of hers was later to prove very important to them as a family in ways then unforseen.

When Vestey's meatworks opened in Darwin in 1917, to supply canned beef for the war effort, Val applied and found work there on the condensers. They lived on a wild two-acre block at Parap, a suburb of Darwin. Their home was crude and a bit small for them, but they extended it themselves when two more children arrived.

Though money was short, the children had a marvellous lifestyle—exploring, hunting, fishing, riding horses, going camping and playing family games. Val built a tennis court using ant-bed for the clay base and Jessie made the net of heavy twine. He and Jessie joined in some of the family favourites like quoits and rounders. Jessie wrote a charming verse about the family at play:

Rounders

The children are playing "rounders"
And I hear them gaily shout
As they play about on the sunlit green
"Over the fence is OUT".

"Over the fence" lies the city,
Where manhood works and strives;
But only a deadened murmur
Reaches the children's lives.

Sheltered from life's temptations,
Free from its care and pain;
I fancy them child-angels
Re-visiting earth again.

And ever I long to join them,
And share in their merry rout;
But I've sent my ball o'er the garden wall
And—"Over the fence is OUT".

Not able to afford transport, "We walked everywhere: down to the circular tank at Vesteys for a swim, to the Oval at Darwin when sports were being held, to the Methodist church for the Band of Hope meetings, to the Town Hall for fancy-dress balls and concerts, to the Don Stadium for the pictures. We never minded the walks; pleasures were all the more keenly enjoyed when they were hard to get, and we certainly took our fill of them". Once again, her wonderfully positive attitude to hardships shines through. This attitude was to sustain her in the dark times that lay ahead.

In 1923, her second son Boyne performed an act of extraordinary bravery. Just eleven, he jumped down a 9 metre-deep well to save the life of his two-year-old brother, Ken, who was drowning in 3 metres of water. Val and Jessie were both very proud parents when Boyne was awarded the Royal Humane Society Medal for bravery. (His sister Betty was awarded a certificate by the same society years later when she dived in and saved the life of a drowning man, John Cubillo, at Rapid Creek.)

Vestey's closed in 1923.

Having loved their time at Anson Bay, the Litchfields decided to apply for a government lease and loan to start a farming and trading enterprise there. Jessie wrote many letters to the Government to argue their case, pointing out social benefits for the area and also that "we can face difficulties boldly and do not need spoon-feeding". The Government turned a deaf ear, except to offer her and her children a fare out of the Territory. This incensed Jessie because her purpose was to help in its development, not to run away.

Fortunately, Val's engineering skills enabled him to find temporary work at the power station. However, when that job also finished, the family were looking down the barrel at possible destitution. Jessie wrote later that it had tugged at her heartstrings whenever she could not adequately feed her family. But this time Val was not always the great help he had been in the past; he appeared to lack energy, suffered from headaches and became a little morose. This was the only period where tensions crept into a marriage that had been extraordinarily happy and Jessie sometimes wrote in letters a little patronisingly about Val's inability to find work. However, the world was heading towards the Great Depression and work had become very hard to come by. This tension was a minor blip compared with the love they shared.

Strong Territorian sentiments were often expressed in Jessie's writings. Here is a quote from *Women's Mirror*, written in 1925:

> Altogether the testing in the Territory is severe, but those who have faith may see the vision of the future, when the land shall be spanned with railways and isolation, neglect and misrepresentation shall be things of the past. In the future we shall see the Northern Territory the glory of Australia, the gateway of the North, the mainstay of the Commonwealth; we shall see miles of docks, scores of mines, hundreds of factories and great aviation hangars...These things will come in our day; but we have a share of the work to do. It is our right and our privilege to prepare the foundation on the stability of which the whole structure will depend.

Visionary articles like these struck a chord with proud Territorians and her personal popularity increased. She stood for council in 1927 but was defeated. "Darwin is not yet ready for a woman to be elected to a position of authority," she concluded. She tried again in 1928 and 1929, finally writing bitterly, "There are still a few survivors from the Stone Age lingering about Darwin, and a large number of these troglodytes absolutely refused to vote for me because I was a woman." This claim was not without foundation and both local newspapers admitted that there had been a large degree of sexual prejudice. The *Northern Territory Times* itself admitted that it thought Jessie would make a brilliant councillor, but that a woman's place was in the home and not dodging about attending to other people's business. The *Standard* agreed wholeheartedly.

Jessie's years of writing were reaping better and better financial rewards, just when her family needed the money most desperately. She wrote increasingly for the two local newspapers and was paid well for her book, *Far North Memories*. Best of all, she became editor of the *Northern Territory Times* in 1930, despite strong local opposition because she was a woman.

Val died soon afterwards, aged 47. The reason for his death was given as "cerebral infarction caused by malignant malaria". Jessie believed it to be the malaria he had contracted at Anson Bay years before that had left a sinister legacy.

Suddenly and unexpectedly alone, Jessie struggled on gamely, bringing up her large family of seven children while still earning a living. She mourned Val over the years and never formed another romantic attachment. She sought some solace in writing nostalgic verse. Here is an insightful excerpt in which she foresees a positive role that Val's death could have in shaping her character:

> I have my dreams. Though lone and drear
> The paths I tread in silence here,
> Yet loss will teach me how to love
> As herbs, when crushed, new fragrance give;
> So from my grief I build anew
> A braver life, more strong and true,
> Nor mourn for what can never be;
> For still one joy is left to me;
> I have my dreams.

Her work as editor was outstanding and, despite the Great Depression, the *Northern Territory Times'* circulation figures improved.

Basically conservative and Territorian, she fought some editorial battles with the leftist *Northern Standard*, the only rival newspaper. The *Standard* began to drop in popularity and had to do something desperate to survive, which it did by purchasing the *Times*, to become the only newspaper in Darwin. This it did in July 1932, and sacked its protagonist Jessie at the same time.

This was not as great a disaster as it would have been several years earlier because she had built up sufficient credibility while editor to act as a reporter for the southern newspapers. This earned her enough to survive on, but only just, as events of national interest were few and far between in the Territory and she was paid only for copy that was published. She would go to the police court in the mornings, and then speak to people down town, sniffing out news. Resourcefully, she would chase up stories by travelling out of town, thereby getting her copy sent away before the other reporters did, who tended to wait in Darwin for the news to come to them. She filled in leisure time by writing novels (all unpublished), corresponding with friends, collecting stamps, taking photographs, acting in plays, playing tennis most evenings and shooting.

An event that captured the world's imagination was the London–Australia Air Race. Reuters had such confidence in Jessie by 1934 that they wanted her to cover it for them unaided, while the other newspapers had two reporters apiece operating in shifts. She was terrified lest she miss anything important. "I was able to hold my own with them, even though they were young men with the latest training and I was just a local who had taught myself the work. My cables reporting the arrival of Scott and Black reached England fifteen minutes before those of the other reporters, and that counts a lot with Reuters."

When the Second World War began, Jessie continued reporting for a living and also involved herself with Red Cross work in a voluntary capacity. Darwin, though, was coming under the threat of bombing and invasion. In a letter of hers in April 1942, we read: "The authorities are insisting on the evacuation of all women and children from Darwin; I have not gone yet and intend to remain here as long as possible." In fact, she moved only when the authorities threatened to pick her up and put her aboard the ship! We can sense her deep disgust at how the evacuation was conducted and its aftermath in this account she wrote:

> Word came from the Commonwealth Government that all civilians were to be compulsorily evacuated from the North, and the women and children were the first to be removed under these orders. Whether the decision for evacuation was a right or a wrong one is still a debatable question; there is no doubt whatever that the method of such evacuation was crude and cruel in the extreme.
>
> Only barest necessities could be taken by the evacuees; everything else had to be left behind; but no arrangements were ever made for the safeguarding of their possessions; apparently, it was not the business of the Commonwealth Government to protect their own people's belongings, which were left to the looter and despoiler.
>
> The evacuees were crammed into ships with unnecessary haste; in one case, eleven women and children had to share a four-berth cabin, and that in December, the hottest and worst month of the year. Food on the boats was insufficient and water, whether by accident or design, was brackish and almost undrinkable. There was no comfort and no consideration shown to these evacuees, who received less help and less consideration from their own government than did the Japanese men and women who were being interned in the southern States: all of their goods accompanied them to the internment camps. The Australian women and children were the ones who suffered most, and were least considered.
>
> Arrived in the southern States, the evacuees were left to fend for themselves! Those who had relatives and friends in the South were the fortunate ones, but there were many whose whole lives had been spent in the Territory, and who had known no other home. Their plight was pitiful; can one wonder that some of them gave up the struggle for existence and simply faded out of life, too sick at heart to carry on any longer?
>
> Very different indeed was the treatment meted out to our evacuees from Hong Kong and Singapore; they received the

utmost assistance from government officials; were granted liberal sustenance, were provided with comfortable accommodation, were found suitable good-paying jobs, and were treated as guests of honour, whom it was a pleasure to serve.

Indeed, Jessie found surviving in the southern cities difficult. Fortunately, all her children were independent and she had only herself to care for, though she struggled with her concerns about them throughout this era of upheaval. For example, Christa, who was eight months pregnant, and her young son Stan, were evacuated to Perth having been given just half an hour to pack. A few days after arriving, Christa gave birth to a second son, Marshall Perron. Jessie's daughter-in-law, Gladys, and grandchildren, were amongst the dangerously overcrowded evacuees on the "hell ship", the *Zealandia*, and they survived on biscuits and water. Jessie's eldest daughter, Betty, experienced the trauma of having her husband killed in the bombing raid on Darwin in 1942. Subsequently Betty joined the Medical Forces and was posted to England. Ken, Jessie's youngest son, lost his wife, not yet nineteen and "a lovely little thing, so helpful and friendly to everyone", to acute appendicitis. Jessie offered to take care of their daughter, Rosemary. Ken, though, did not avail himself of her offer and married again in 1943.

Jessie took a series of low-paying jobs in the South, including a four-month stint as "Assistant Clerk in a temporary capacity" in Bathurst, and selling stationery. But she was finding mobility difficult now and began to walk longish distances with the aid of a cane, having become quite lame in one leg. She blamed the forced evacuation for her lameness but no doubt being overweight contributed to its severity. Finally she bought the Roberta Library, a small business that by sheer hard work she worked up into a profitable enterprise.

At war's end Jessie, now in her early sixties, could well have opted to remain in the South because her business was doing well. Besides, she could no longer get about sufficiently to be a reporter and would have to transport her Roberta Library to Darwin and reopen it there, an enormous challenge in war-ravaged Darwin.

Her heart, though, had never left the Territory and she had an abiding distaste for Australian cities apart from Darwin, as can be seen in her personifications in a strange little sketch:

> Melbourne is a great, sprawling harridan; a blowsy old woman, hard and vulgar, hiding her natural evil under a too-short cloak of respectability. Please keep a thin veneer of whitewash over the stinking cesspools of the city, but never clean them out, for then the stench might spread abroad.
>
> Sydney is a laughing hoyden who doesn't care. Too happy to be coarse and common, she calls you to share her green gardens and surf beaches with her. She gets away with anything by her very freedom.
>
> Brisbane is a country town trying to ape the cities and succeeds only in being ridiculous.

She began a campaign before leaving Sydney by writing to the Government, and anyone else who would listen, for fair compensation to be given Darwinites whose homes had been destroyed by bombs or looters. She also produced several visionary and detailed documents for the replanning of Darwin because "we could make Darwin the most beautiful city in Australia; but it needs careful planning… by folk who build with their hearts as well as with their heads and their hands". She was dismissed in a patronising fashion by many to whom she appealed. She then suggested Darwinites should sit on committees that were replanning the city, and again her appeal was dismissed. Now very frustrated, Jessie became more radical in the opinions she expressed. Her writings after the war hardened in tone and her calls for self-government for the Territory became more strident:

> We need self-government; the right to run our own affairs as WE think best and not as Canberra orders; we need a Member in Parliament who has not only a voice, but a vote… We object to control by Canberra; where every change of parliamentary power means a change in the policy by which the territory is controlled; we want the right to elect our own government, composed of the folk whom we know and trust; in short, we want a square deal: shall we ever get it?

Nor had Jessie simply returned to Darwin at war's end as the city was still under the control of the military. Besides, her son Boyne wrote to her telling her to wait because he and his family had not been allowed to proceed further than Pine Creek, and the conditions there left much to be desired. The population there grew daily with frustrated returnees who were forced to wait also. Boyne and his family of three children, soon to become four, lived in a crude tin shed at Pine Creek for two interminable years before being allowed home to Darwin in 1946.

The Darwin that greeted Jessie shocked her because it had been savaged more than she had anticipated. Barbed wire, paper and pieces of wrecked furniture were strewn everywhere. Many of the old landmarks were bomb-wrecked shells, the central Post Office being one example. Her own home had escaped the bombing but not the looting. She entered, hoping to find some of her goods and chattels intact, but nothing of value remained. She could understand her valuable stamp collection being stolen, but even her extensive collection of press cuttings had gone. So had photograph albums, boxes of personal letters and autographed copies of books. Exhausted and close to tears, she took some minutes to gather herself together. Then she set her mouth, and her heart. Like the phoenix, she was determined to rise out of the ashes. Once again, she displayed the pioneering spirit at its best.

After a gigantic struggle in a Darwin where building materials were like gold, Jessie designed and built a shop and home on a block in Mitchell Street. Her years of helping Val build and extend the different homes they had lived in stood her in good stead. The finished premises were tidy and smart; the front was of cypress pine and fibrolite with two show windows and a ripple glass door. (Indeed, it won a prize for its presentation during a competition to mark the Coronation of Queen Elizabeth in 1953.) Inside was a large showroom where she opened her Roberta Library. She sold cards, comics, stamps, books, dress patterns and general stationery as well as operating as a library. Behind the shop were her private rooms including a bedroom, office, kitchen-dining room and shower room.

A further measure of Jessie's greatness lies in the way she sent parcels of food to their erstwhile enemies in Germany and Eastern Europe. She did this from 1947 to 1949 despite her own shortages and financial struggles. Here are just a couple of excerpts from among grateful letters of appreciation:

> Julius Meier from Frankfurt, Germany, on 1.10.1949:
> I have lost my home in the war by bombs from the Royal Air Force"…and later, "To my great pleasure I can inform you that I got, a few days ago, your very nice gift parcel—the last you sent. It contains many very nice things and my family will use it with much happiness.

> Dusau Pacic from Beograd, Yugoslavia, on 14.7.49:
> You mention in your letter that you have sent three parcels till now. I am sorry, but I have received only one… It is very kind of you and we really need the cocao, coffee, milk, sugar, etc. but as I have mentioned I cannot pay you—only if you wish stamps.

Her business had become quite profitable by 1951 and Jessie turned her eyes once more to contesting an election, this time standing as an independent for the federal seat in Canberra. Aged 68 and unable to move around without great effort, she hired a taxi to carry her for 5000 kilometres of campaigning around the Territory. Her main platform was the need for self-government, allied to the need for land reform and an improved communication network. She polled well but failed in her bid, blaming once again the fact that she was a woman. In fact, it was 1960 before a woman, Lyn Berlowitz, won any election in the Territory.

Feisty as ever, Jessie continued to promote her favourite issues vigorously. Fittingly, it was her grandson, Marshall Perron, who was Treasurer when the Territory won self-government in 1978 and who would later become its Chief Minister.

Meanwhile, her influence on Flynn's work came full circle when Fred McKay became the new Superintendent of the AIM. Fred visited her regularly and consulted with her because the AIM had nursing homes in the Territory and plans for other mission work. "I was struck by her intelligence and by her Christian commitment. She dressed like a businesswoman and was always welcoming and affable. Her arms were tanned and her face had been barked by the sun. Her eyes were clear and she fixed you with an unblinking, penetrating gaze."

More sedentary now, Jessie continued with her writing, photography and a new hobby—cats. She won awards for all three at the Darwin Show.

In 1953, Jessie was at last accorded recognition for the contribution she had made to the Territory when she was awarded the Coronation Medal. Another honour followed in 1955 when she was appointed as a Justice of the Peace for the Northern Territory, the first woman to be so honoured.

Jessie and the Roberta had become a bit of a gathering place for the literary minded. She had long believed that a magazine of quality would help to promote the Territory in the South and encourage tourism, and told her visitors so. She discussed this idea in depth with a like-minded freelance writer, Glenville Pike, who visited her at the Roberta Library. He decided to run with the concept and in 1954 launched the *North Australian Monthly*, with Jessie as assistant editor. She was right in her element again and wrote prolifically about Darwin and the North in general. The magazine was a success.

Then in 1956, aged 73, she decided to take a holiday "Down South". She visited friends and family in Brisbane and Sydney and then went to Canberra, where she was honoured with a seat on the floor of the House. Moving on, she stayed in Melbourne in the home of her cousin and good friend, J.K. Moir. He returned one evening to find her on the kitchen floor, face downwards. She had died from a heart attack.

On July 19th 1956, there was a moving memorial service in the same church in Knucky Street, Darwin, in which she had been married in 1907 and of which she had been so faithful a member over many years. It was the last service to be held in that church before the building of a new one. The following evening boasted a glorious sunset and her ashes were scattered from an aeroplane over an area she had grown to love, the Darwin Harbour and surrounds.

Flynn's Mentors

Jeannie Gunn and Jessie Litchfield

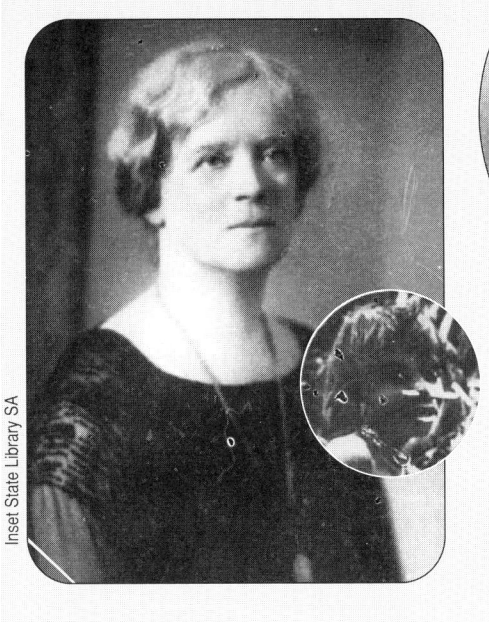

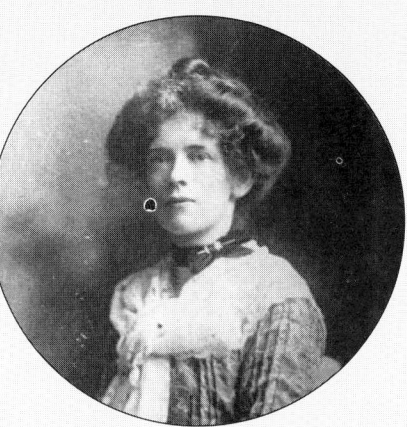

Above: The woman with whom Aeneas Gunn fell in love - Jeannie before she went to Elsey.

Left: The famous author, by this time widowed, wearing the pendant given her by Bett-Bett (inset), Jeannie's inspiration for "The Little Black Princess".

Right: Although lame after her enforced evacuation from Darwin in 1942, Jessie campaigned vigorously for the things about which she felt passionate. She is holding the camera that as a journalist she carried everywhere.

Left: It's 1953 and Jessie Litchfield proudly wears her coronation medal.

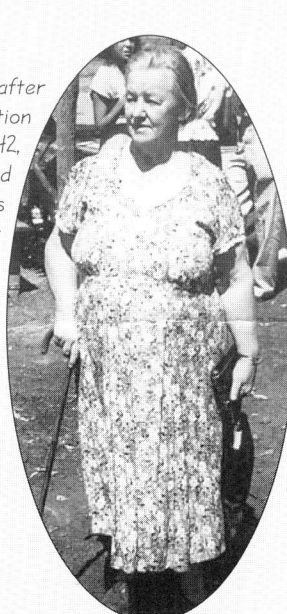

Pioneering Nurses

From top: Sister Jean Finlayson.

Myrtle Villa in Alice Springs, 1916, where Jean Finlayson lived and conducted her clinics.

Jean Finlayson's first camp en route to Alice Springs in 1915

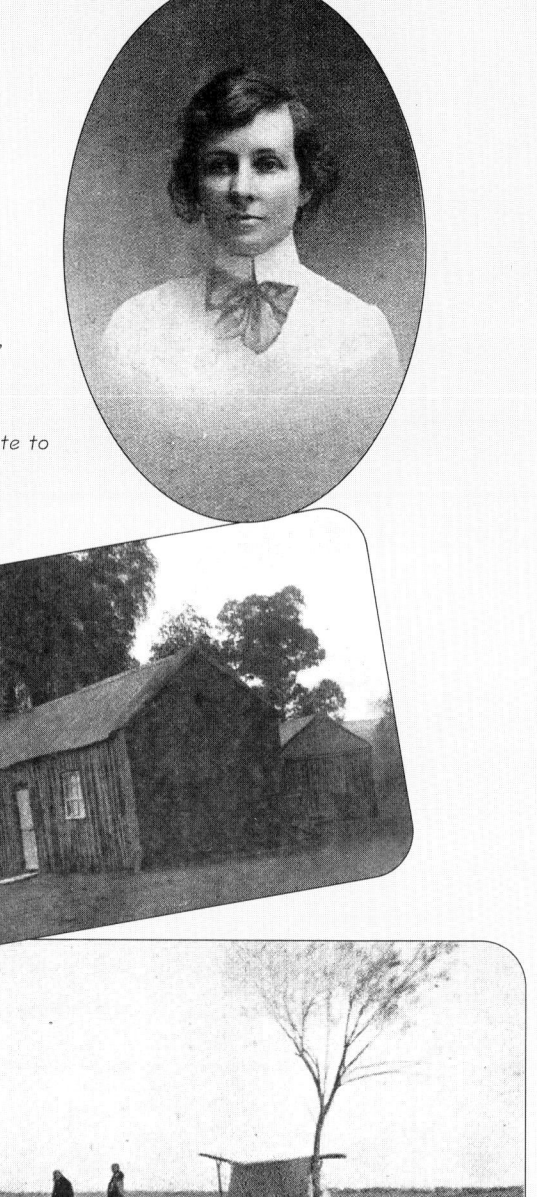

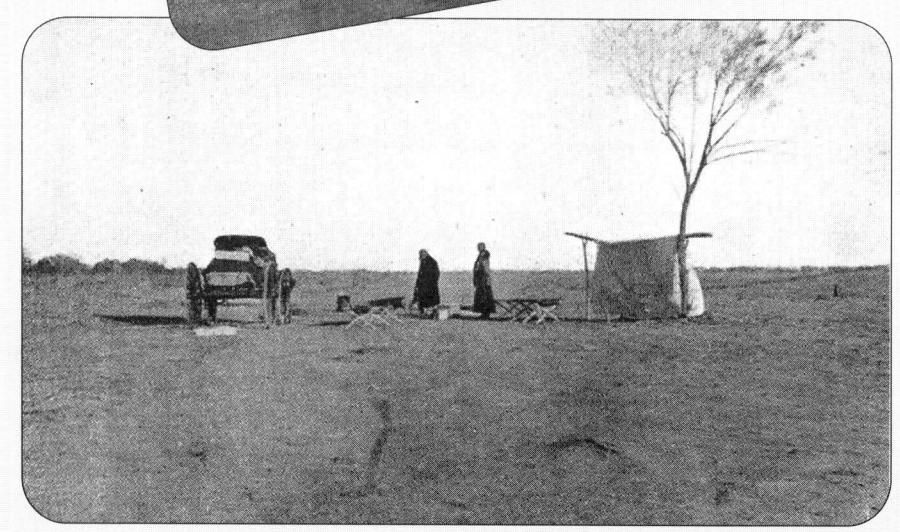

Left: Jean Finlayson successfully treated these children for exposure. They had run away from the Bungalow and were discovered buried up to their necks in sand to escape the fierce Central Australian sun - a stratagem employed by many Aboriginal groups living in the arid zone.

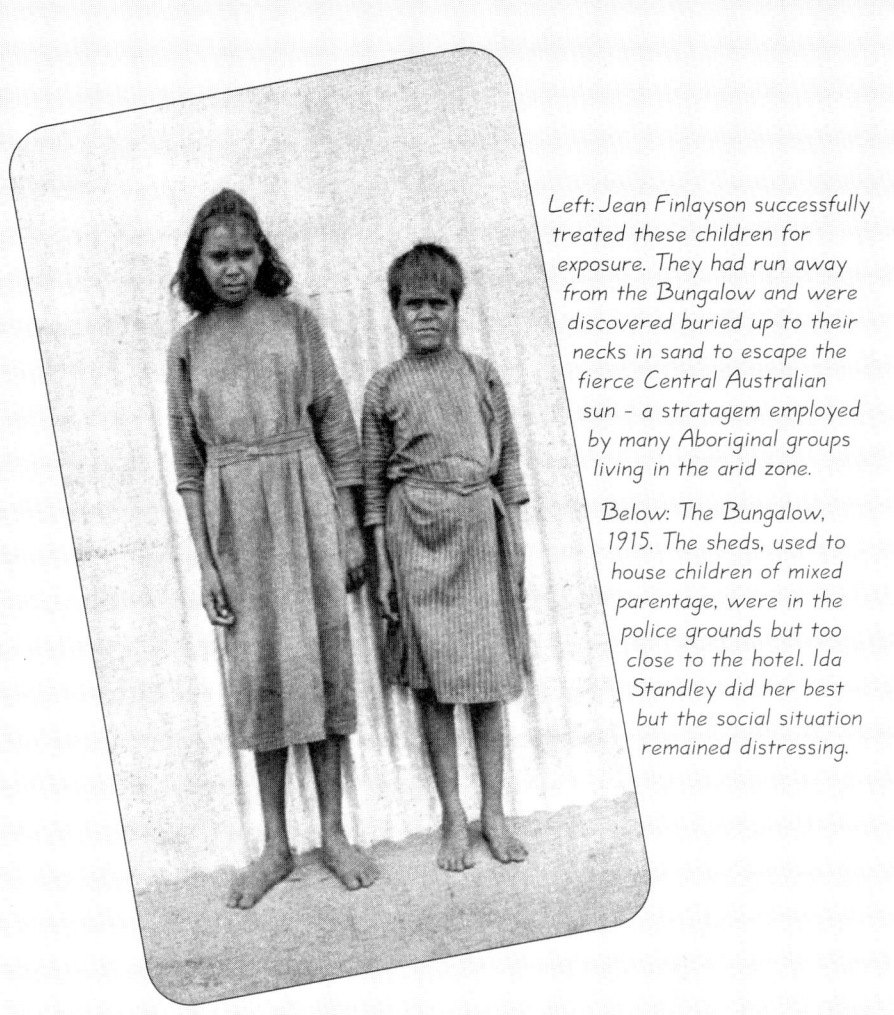

Below: The Bungalow, 1915. The sheds, used to house children of mixed parentage, were in the police grounds but too close to the hotel. Ida Standley did her best but the social situation remained distressing.

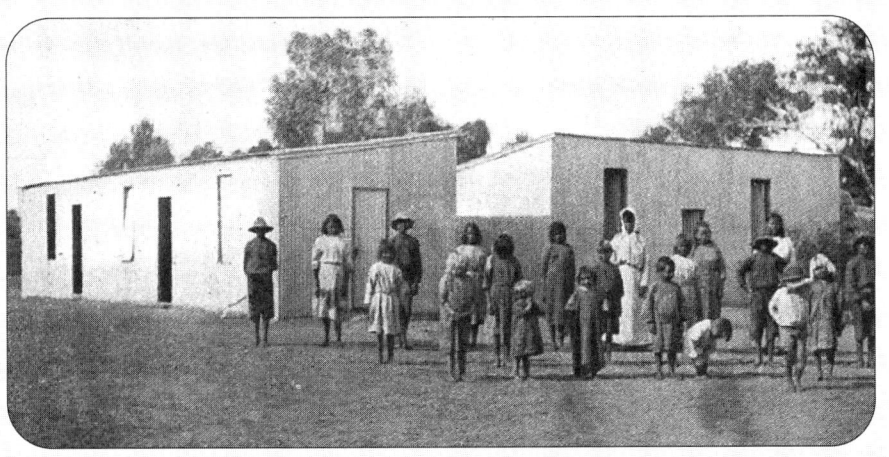

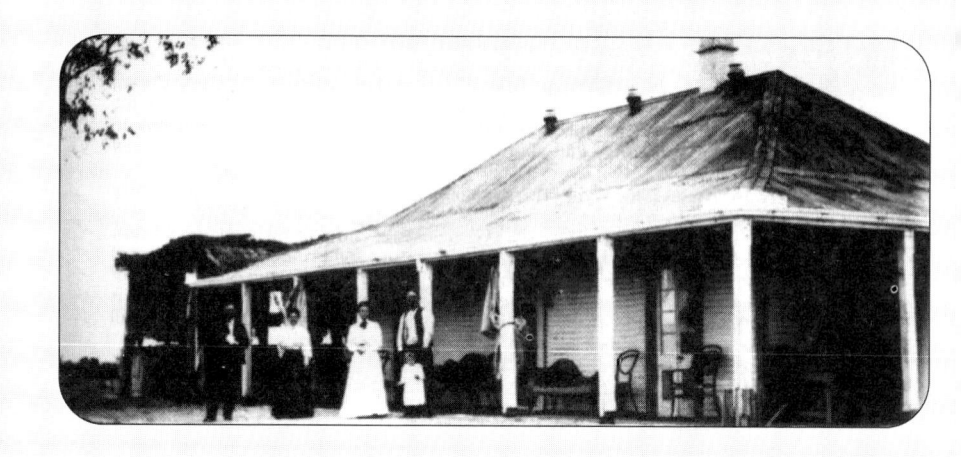

Above: Innamincka station homestead where Minnie Kinnear nursed the sick on the verandah and conducted clinics in the outbuildings.

Below from left: John Flynn, Minnie Kinnear, Elsie Coultas - an ardent supporter of the AIM - and Reverend Armour. The photo was taken at Beltana in 1919 when Minnie was matron of its new AIM hospital.

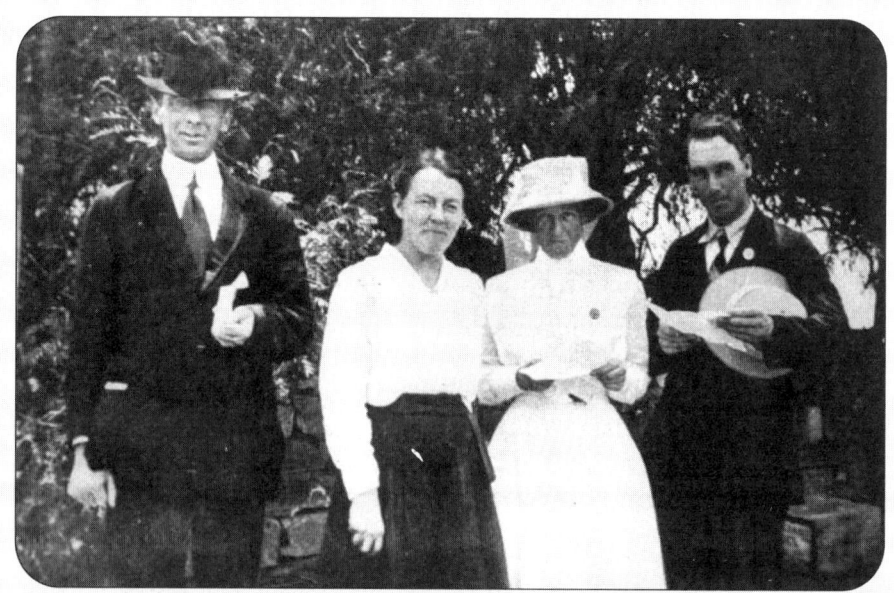

State Library SA

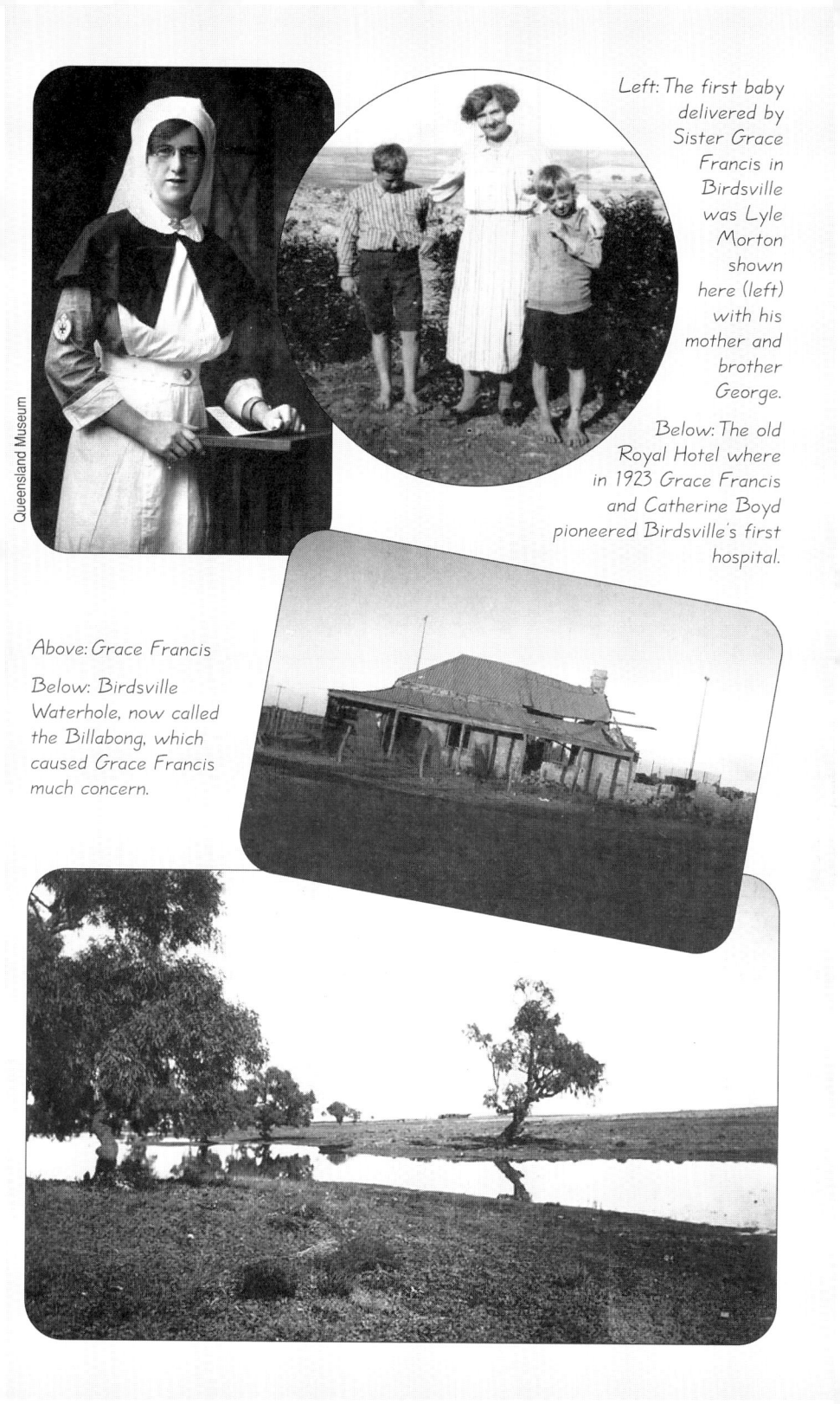

Left: The first baby delivered by Sister Grace Francis in Birdsville was Lyle Morton shown here (left) with his mother and brother George.

Below: The old Royal Hotel where in 1923 Grace Francis and Catherine Boyd pioneered Birdsville's first hospital.

Above: Grace Francis

Below: Birdsville Waterhole, now called the Billabong, which caused Grace Francis much concern.

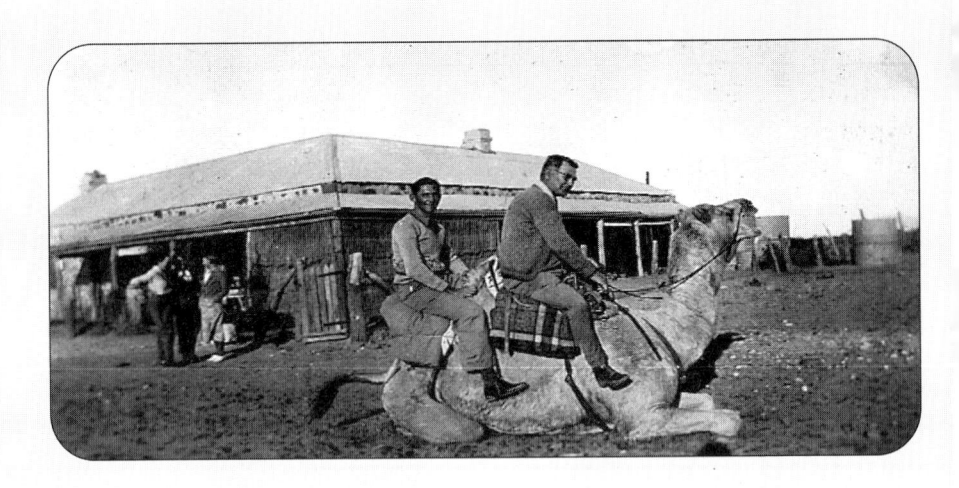

Above: Lou Reese transported Sisters Grace Francis and Catherine Boyd on the last leg of their journey to Birdsville and was a helpful friend to a succession of nurses. Here he is in 1936 in front of the Brisbane Home giving Fred McKay (at rear) a camel ride.

Below: Grace Francis and Catherine Boyd return to Birdsville in 1953 for the dedication of the new hospital, its predecessor having been destroyed by fire in 1951. Catherine Boyd talks to the hero of the fire, Sister Mona Henry (left), while Grace Francis chats to Sister Mary Chenoweth and Sister Beth Forrest listens in.

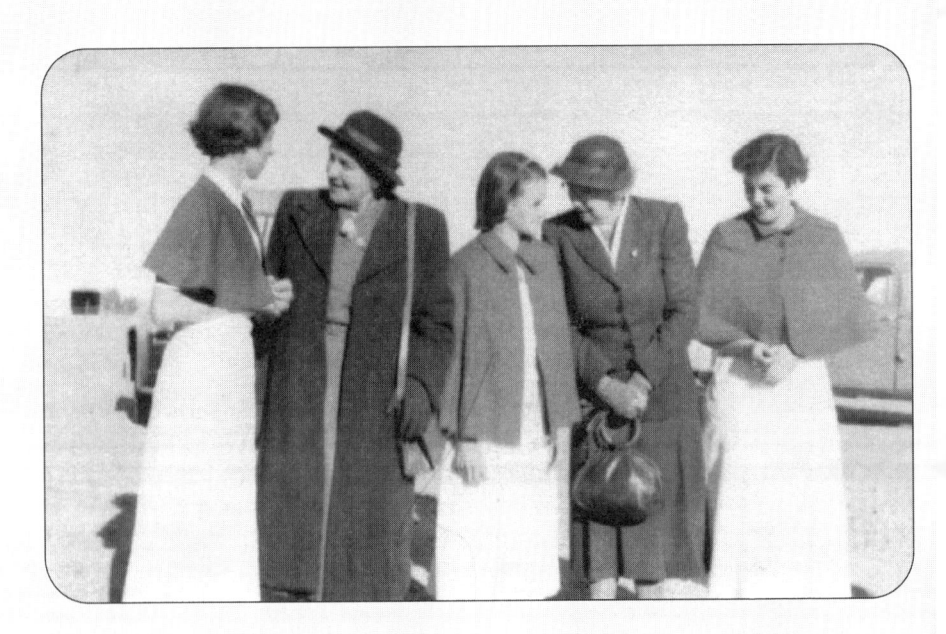

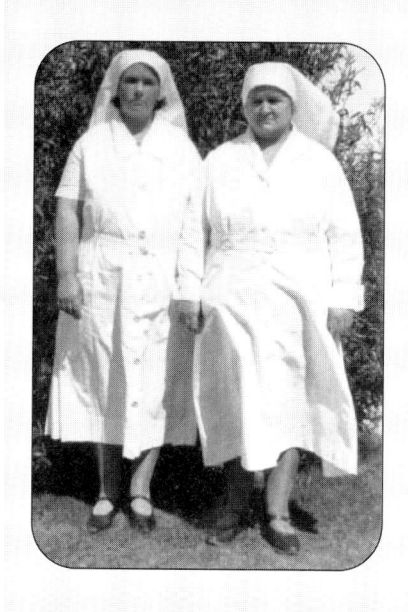

The Inglis Sisters

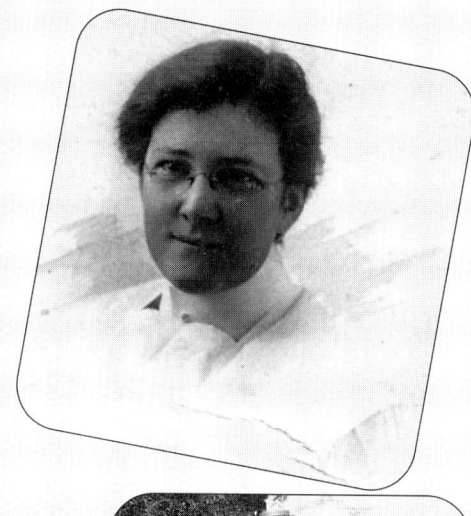

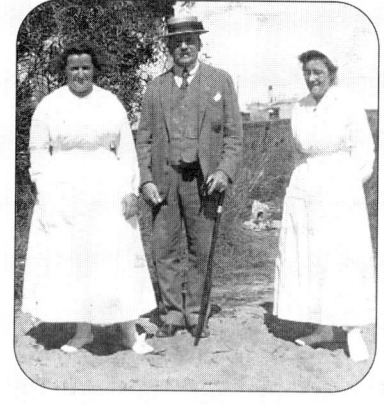

Clockwise from top left: Sister Elsie Sim (left) and Nance. Cousins and lifetime friends, they served together at Beltana.

Nell Inglis in uniform.

Nance and Nell with the Governor of WA. VIPs and politicians liked being photographed at AIM hospitals.

Nance (left), as matron of Warrawee, led a happy staff.

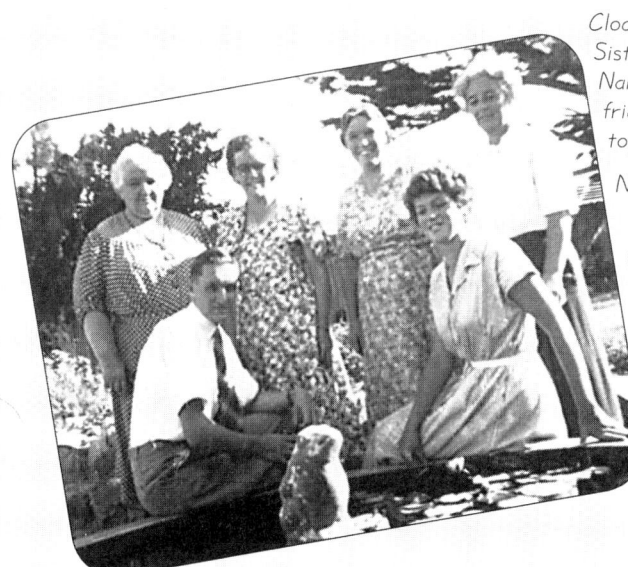

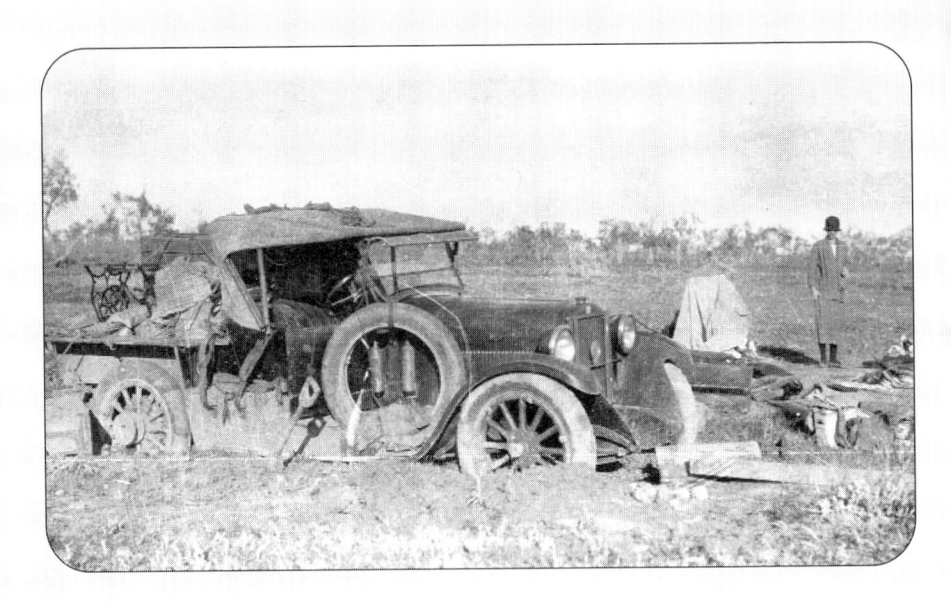

Above: John Flynn bogged in May 1926 while taking Sisters Ina Pope and Ellen Small to Alice Springs. They detoured to rescue a man at Horseshoe Bend, rushing him to Oodnadatta in time to catch the southbound train to Port Augusta and a life-saving operation. Meanwhile, heavy rains had turned the "road" to slush.

"Daily they bandaged Flynn's bloodied hands". Lean and smiling, John Flynn stands between Ellen Small and Ina Pope on 26th June 1926. The occasion was the opening of the nursing home he built at Alice Springs

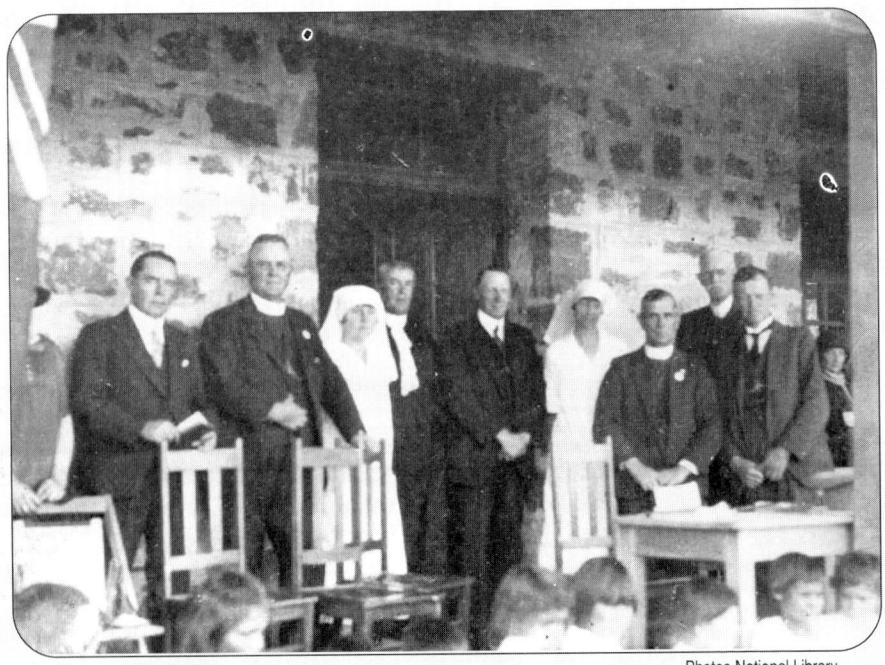

Photos National Library

Most of her estate was left to the Melbourne Bread and Cheese Club. She wished them to administer an annual award in an effort to foster good literature: "It is to encourage a healthy, happy Australian spirit and to advance the simple virtues of loyalty and courage." This encapsulated her own approach to life. And where did that approach come from? The eulogy in the *North Australian Weekly* of September 1956 suggested this answer:

> We may be sure that the secret of her excellent example in life and of her high standard of citizenship is to be found in the Christian faith she cherished.

Another eulogy came from her former teacher, Dame Mary Gilmore, who had this to say about Jessie:

> In Northern Australia in and beyond Darwin she was a builder, an influence and a historian. Her interest never dulled and her spirit never failed. She personified the true Territorian. Her passing was a loss to the Australian people.

Fred McKay, many years later, said, "I have always believed that Jeannie Gunn and Jessie Litchfield were the two women who most influenced Flynn's thinking. He would visit them and discuss his plans with them. They both had a significant input into all that Flynn achieved."

And so the pages that follow are partly their legacy, these two great pioneering women, because they inspired Flynn to reach out to attempt the impossible. Both were extraordinarily positive in their advice despite their own personal tragedies and difficulties. Thus they lead the parade of great women that supported him. And just behind these two stride heroic nurses, of whom we read next.

4

Nurses Without Hospitals—
Jean Finlayson and Minnie Kinnear

The great Sister Latto Bett, known as "The Little Angel of the North", told Flynn as early as 1913 that she intended to serve in the war that was approaching in Europe. "There I'll be able to help hundreds each week," she explained. This meant that Flynn's first cottage hospital at Oodnadatta would be left without a nurse in attendance, unless he could find a replacement.

How can you replace a legend? For four years the "little Sister" had been nurse, teacher, preacher, confidante, sometimes doctor and always friend to the community. The children she gave correspondence lessons to, or were in her lively Sunday School, the young women she helped make dresses in city fashions, the mothers she counselled, the elderly she visited, the men whose health she restored—all these and many more loved her. Her dedication was extraordinary. Even her "holidays" had been spent largely assisting in operating theatres and dental clinics to learn more so that she could help more.

Flynn cast around desperately before finding Sister Jean Finlayson, a triple-certificated Sister who was also a Deaconess and therefore well able to replace Sister Bett in the holding of church services and Sunday School. But how well would she do in looking after the rough, tough "bushies" that Sister Bett had dealt with so expertly? Much would depend upon her personality.

The train arrived in Oodnadatta once a fortnight on a Friday. As "Oodna" was the railhead, it would turn around and return to Adelaide the following Tuesday. Jean arrived hot, tired and dusty late one night in February 1914 and was surprised to find half the town on the platform. Sister Bett and Bruce Plowman, Flynn's first and great Patrol Padre, introduced her around. She was breathless, flushed and excited by the warm welcome she received. Despite the late hour, she was given a good meal and then shown around the premises. Jean was delighted by the compact and efficient little hospital that Flynn had built. She then went to bed. Having just three full days to learn the ropes from Sister Bett, she would need to be alert the following day.

Sister Bett woke her early with a plate of steaming breakfast and a bundle of letters. She then left Jean alone to get up.

Jean looked out the window and was struck by the long camel train that wound its way out the village. It had collected the mail and much else off the train already and was now the main system of transport for all destinations north. In the course of time, she would attend to the "Afghan" cameleers. (She remarked later: "The Afghans were good patients and their teeth easy to pull, unlike the Aborigines whose teeth only dislodged with a great struggle.")

It was a blur of activity until Sister Bett left. Jean, who had lived a protected life in Melbourne, was surprised by the rough repartee between the Little Sister and some of the bushmen.

"I taught her all she knows, didn't I, Jack? Came out to the bush knowing nothing, didn't she?" This was the "Grumpy Saint" baiting her. Plowman, who saw the heart of gold beneath a rough exterior, gave him that nickname.

"Yes, thank you so much for your kindness. You have been a wonderful teacher and expert in medical things. Your explanation about orthodontics was most helpful."

"There she goes again, talking city stuff. I don't think we succeeded with her after all."

This banter was obviously affectionate and never crude, but it left Jean feeling uneasy because her own personality was a lot more reserved. Would she be able to get along with these men well enough for them to respect her? Would her nursing services be rejected if she were to be rejected? And what about the church services she must hold, would they be attended?

In his book, *The Man From Oodnadatta*, which has recently been updated by his daughter Jean Whitla, Bruce Plowman has left us a brilliant description of what happened next:

> Sunday night—only one clear day before the Little Sister was to leave. Bushmen from far and near had gathered for the occasion. It was late when black-bearded Jack drew the Padre [Plowman himself] aside and suggested a walk. Next

morning Jack was to make the speech of farewell and present the bushmen's parting gift.

"Don't know how I'm going to make a speech tomorrow," he said as he halted beside a fence.

Quite abruptly he sank on his haunches with his back to the fence and began playing nervously with a stone. "It's damnable!" he said at last, as if speaking to himself. The other kept silent, not knowing what comment to make.

Presently, Jack began to talk. Taking his hearer back to the time of his accident, he recounted all that the Little Sister had done for him. In vividly illuminating words he told the story of the long fight in the silent ward; of the dreary days and the sleepless nights of agony; of his declining hold on life and his desire that all would be speedily over; of his unutterable longing for rest; of the Little Sister's hopeless task and her heroic unwillingness to accept defeat.

"There was one night…" The aggressive bushman's voice was low and shaky. His companion dared not look in his face for fear of discovering the tears, which he himself felt hardly able to control. "…one night when I knew I was going to die, and she knew I was going to die; and I would have died, only she wouldn't let me."

The farewell on the Hostel lawn next morning was memorable. About forty men from the township and from stations hundreds of miles apart made up the crowd. Among them was the six-foot-six bushman who had recently been to church after so long an absence.

The Little Sister–five feet tall and weighing seven stone [45 kg]–stood white-costumed in the sunlight before them all. Never before had she looked so tiny. But, gallant little soul, she showed no sign of the emotion which possessed her; confident and serene, she awaited the ordeal.

For four years she had compelled the respect of these men, for the religion and morals that she represented. She had won their high regard; and, departing, would maintain the same relationship.

Jack started to make a speech; broke down; swallowed hard at a choking lump in his throat; pushed the roll of cheques and notes into the Little Sister's hand; brushed his hand across his eyes; and backed into the crowd.

At the same moment, the Grumpy Saint shook his head as if angry with his friend; turned on his heel and strode off as if disgusted with the whole proceeding. Only the stifled sob which shook his sturdy frame, and the tears flowing down his cheeks, betrayed his true feelings.

Jean, watching this, realised sharply how difficult it was going to be to fill Sister Bett's shoes. And when she left one day, would there be a crowd of grateful bushmen to farewell her? Plowman describes what happened next:

> The new Sister did not get time to sit in idleness after the departure of her predecessor. There was a knock on the side door.
>
> "Oh, Sister," said an agitated mother, "would you mind coming in to have a look at a baby? I don't know what's the matter with her."
>
> Sister went in and examined the baby, a beautiful girl child of about ten months. Her little body was splendidly formed and well nourished, and there seemed to be nothing wrong except that her eyes were lifeless and her temperature above normal.
>
> "What happened to her?"
>
> The mother shook her head. "Nothing's happened to her that I know of. She was all right early this morning. She took her breakfast and enjoyed her bath, and went to sleep like she always does. Later on I thought I heard her whimpering and went to the bedroom, and she was like she is now."
>
> The Sister asked many questions but could obtain no clue as to the baby's strange illness. Unfortunately, the doctor was away. [He was a railways doctor, and often out of town in the railway camps.]
>
> "I think I had better take baby into the Hostel where I can watch her," Sister said; and took the baby with her and laid her on a white cot in the big ward.
>
> "Wish I had some ice!" the Sister said to the Padre, who had called to see her and found her fanning the wee naked body. "I've got to get this child's temperature down somehow. It's gone up alarmingly. I've tried everything I know and can't reduce it. It is simply burning her up."

The temperature would not come down; the day was hot; and the Sister kept on fanning.

"Let me take a turn while you have a spell, Sister."

She shook her head. "I daren't. She's too ill. I'll have to watch her every moment if I'm to save her. I would never forgive myself if any change came and I was not on the spot to take advantage of it."

The day passed slowly.

For odd minutes, she let the mother take the fan, when some necessary duty called her away, but returned and took over as quickly as possible. She had taken no dinner, she took no tea; and still she fanned, while the baby's life steadily burned out.

Late that night the baby died. On its left elbow a tiny bruise, which the mother could not account for, was the only mark on its otherwise perfect little body.

The Sister's fan slowed and stopped. Tears of grief and disappointment welled in her eyes as her tired arm sank to her side. For eleven hours she had stood beside the cot trying to ward off death with a moving fan.

Eleven hours! Try it for eleven minutes and see how your arm aches. Eleven hours—and then failure.

The Sister went to bed that night heavy of heart and weary of body.

Some things are not spectacular; but they are none the less heroic.

Jean had many successes, but heart-rending failures also. Here is her own description of one case taken from a little book she wrote, *Life and Journeyings in Central Australia*:

> I recall the case of another little child, just a mite a few days old; with but slight warning its newly-given life passed out. And being an only son, its life had been very precious.
>
> The sick and troubled mother asked me to bury her babe. Now, it had never occurred to me that I might ever be called upon to perform such a service. [But fortunately she remembered that John Flynn had written out a burial service in his book, *The Bushman's Companion*.]
>
> The Smith and Carpenter prepared a tiny white casket in which we placed the sleeping babe. The old

grandmother plucked from her little cottage garden such flowers that she had.

Covered by a rug, the little casket was conveyed in a spring cart. I, accompanied by the other two women, followed in a buggy to some little distance from the village to the burial ground, marked only by broken fences and a few mounds of earth.

At the graveside we were met by a young man, hat in hand, leaning upon a shovel.

Using the reins from the horse, this man with the help of the driver, lowered the little casket into its resting place.

Out in that desert place, with the wind howling through the oaks, we five, half-blinded by the flying sand, stood around while I read the burial service from *The Bushman's Companion*.

Through acts such as these, Jean soon established a reputation as a fine, dedicated and compassionate nurse. Within months she reported that she had treated over 400 patients in a short space of time, was suffering from lack of sleep and needed some way to keep her food cool because "the butter is oil". She saved many lives and won the respect of the community.

On those occasions that the railways doctor was in Oodna, she worked alongside him. She described one such case, involving Pat Byrne who had had his arm ripped off when it caught in a bore pump. Dr Abbott met the patient at Hamilton and accompanied him down to Oodnadatta. Jean reported:

> As we have only one ward and that was occupied by a lady and her baby, I was obliged to turn my sitting room into a ward and operating room. Doctor Abbott amputated the arm below the elbow. As the accident happened four days before, the arm was in a shocking condition and the wound will be some time in healing.

With her careful nursing, cleaning and protection of the wound, the arm healed. When Parol Padre Skipper Partridge met him three years later, Pat was healthy and active and running a store at Charlotte Waters.

By nature reserved, Jean did not make friends easily in the same way that Sister Bett had, and attendances at Sunday services, and even in the Sunday School, fell away a little. However, she remained aware that Flynn's concept was that the Hostel should become a community centre and do social and spiritual work as well as medical, so she made an effort:

> I sent an invitation one evening to a lot of drovers and stockmen to come to the Hostel and have a little singing. And if they had not an organist amongst them, I would play.
> They accepted with alacrity, and in a short time all trooped along in their shirtsleeves and riding attire: modest, shy boys all. Still, a lady had invited them, so they came.
> One loves these brave boys, with their sunburnt, smiling faces, fine physique and courteous manner.

Her love of children was well known and she wrote to some and sent presents to others, some of whom she had never met. Elsa Johannsen was living at "Deep Well station, near Alice Springs" in May 1915. Elsa wrote to Flynn that when Plowman unpacked the boxes on his camel Doctor, he produced a doll for her that Sister Jean Finlayson had sent: "I took its bonnet off, and put on it a wreath I made from the leaves of the pepper tree, and it looked nearly like a bride". For isolated children like Elsa, Jean's presents were a tremendous thrill.

Jean and Flynn maintained a regular correspondence. Jean's letters show her to be professional, blunt and a bit critical of others. Flynn's letters show that he was already looking further north towards Alice Springs, because he had travelled there in 1913 and had found a pressing need for medical help. His letters and writings often mentioned these same needs. For example, he quoted a copy of a letter he had received from a pioneer in the North in his *Inlander* magazine, showing how hard confinements were. The husband wrote, "I had to attend to everything myself" and "should any more children come along, I suppose I will have to do the same again". Flynn noted that this man was typical of most men north of Oodnadatta at that time—"a poor man pulling hard against the stream"—because there were few rich cattlemen or miners, but hundreds of battlers.

In his letters to Jean he expressed his concerns for the North more and more stridently. He obviously hoped she might volunteer to fill the role he had first suggested in his 1912 report, that a Nurse–Deaconess be stationed at Alice Springs.

He had unexpected allies in his promptings, the first teacher in the Centre, Ida Standley, and the agitator who had brought her there, Sam Nicker. When Sam had been in Adelaide in 1913 for treatment to an infected eye, that he lost, he had lobbied the Federal Minister for Education for a school in Alice Springs, and he won. Ida Standley had been appointed and spent time with Jean Finlayson in Oodnadatta in 1914 on her way to Alice Springs. She was described to Flynn by Spicer, his friend in the telegraph office at Alice Springs, to be "a woman of mature age and kindly and sensible in her outlook on life". She was 45 years old and had left a husband and children behind.

Arriving at Alice Springs, Ida was appalled how primitive conditions were in the Centre, medically speaking. Soon after her arrival both she and Sam Nicker began writing to Jean to prompt her to come North. Ida, especially, painted a relatively rosy picture:

> If it were not for the dear ones left behind [her husband and children] I should be quite happy. Mr and Mrs Stott [with whom she boarded] are so good to me. I have a large airy bedroom all to myself and a delightful little schoolroom which I also use as a sitting room. Come and join me as soon as possible… I know that you would just love it here.

Ida had other concerns also, of which she wrote to Jean. One was the sad and neglected mixed-race population of the North. A compassionate woman, she described their plight:

> The half-caste girl who remains with the tribe anywhere in the vicinity of a civilised settlement has one inevitable destiny, and that the most degraded… She runs the risk when the time and opportunity are favourable of being actually sold by her tribal relatives for prostitution or taken away by force by some unscrupulous man who keeps her just as long as he cares to.

Jean was hesitant and non-committal in her replies to Ida and to Flynn regarding a move to Alice Springs. But as the months went by, various cases from the primitive North disturbed her also. Regarding confinements, she wrote to Flynn about a Mrs Bloomfield who had her baby without a midwife and "It was three days before that poor woman had the attention of another white woman. The baby died later on. Don't know about the mother's health".

But it was not only maternity cases in the Centre that concerned Jean:

> During the intense heat of February, as I sat one day beneath the shelter of my veranda writing letters and doing battle with flies, an Aboriginal boy opened the gate and handed me a telegram. On opening it I found that it had been sent from a telegraph station 350 miles to the north. "Please send lotion for sore eyes, infected from flies. Urgent" I looked at my watch; yes, I had missed the north mail [by coach and camel] by just two hours, and there would not be another for two weeks, and then it would take eleven days more to get there – in all, twenty-five days.
>
> Going at once to the telegraph station, I wired to the man that his message had come too late, and gave instructions regarding treatment of the eye – there being no doctor in the village at that time.
>
> Returning to the dispensary, I made up a parcel of the necessary lotion and dressings, and kept them ready to hand to the first man that I could find going north who might overtake the mail.
>
> On receiving my reply, the man decided to set out at once on the journey south, as fast as horses could bring him over all those miles of dry country, troubled all the way by the intense heat, flies and dust. This took him eleven days to accomplish, and when he at last arrived it was found that the eye had burst, and there was little to do beyond sending him on the further 688 miles to Adelaide, for an operation, by the first cattle train going south.

These long delays before medicine reached Inlanders reminds us of Flynn's tongue-in-cheek comment when replying to the notion that the Overland Telegraph had made medical facilities better in the bush. He wrote: "you can call up a doctor in Adelaide, get his advice by wire, and take his medicine by imagination".

One of Jean's letters to Flynn stirred him. He simply had to do something! He quoted directly from it in the 1914 General Assembly of the Presbyterian Church:

> The baby from Alice Springs was one year and nine months old. It was the most shocking thing that I have seen. The jaw had been either fractured or dislocated. Its whole head and face was black, and the mouth fixed wide open; the eyes right out of the head, and the child unconscious…. It is a good case for Alice Springs [to have a hospital] as, if there had been a nurse near, it could never have got into that condition.

Flynn then appealed to the Assembly for something to be done to relieve such terrible sufferings. "By the blackened face of that poor child, and the agonised heart of its weary mother, for it must have taken EIGHT DAYS for the parents to reach the hospital, I urge you to roll back the shame of years by doing generously what the nation has been too indifferent even to discuss seriously."

However, the war in Europe had begun and caution regarding monetary outlay was the order of the day. Flynn could not convince his Board to build a nursing home in Alice Springs despite hearing further examples of suffering there. He could stand it no longer and turned to Jean, suggesting more urgently that she go and pioneer a nursing outstation in Alice Springs. Flynn knew how well she had served at Oodnadatta and believed that she could succeed further north.

Finally, she could delay a decision no longer:

> A definite request came to me from the Superintendent: "Would I go to Alice Springs and just live there for one year, then report as to conditions and advisability of building a Nursing Home in this little settlement in the heart of the MacDonnell Ranges?"
>
> After much correspondence, it was decided that I should go. And in due time arrangements were made for my stay there—very inadequate arrangements, but the best that could be done.

> I would go in the interests of the sick.
> Those in the North urged me to go, while many others about me urged me, in my own interest, not to go. However, there was only one way of finding out what we wished to know, and I held to my original decision to make the attempt.

Ida Standley was living temporarily with policeman Stott and his wife. She made arrangements that Jean might also stay with them for a short time, so that she would at least have shelter to begin with. Sergeant Robert Stott was also keen for Jean to come because he or his wife Agnes often had to pull teeth, set broken limbs or tend the sick, in the absence of anyone else. Jean would help to relieve their burden.

Jean went knowing that she would have no hospital and no doctor to help, nor pharmacist, nor anywhere permanent to live. She had served for eighteen months already in Oodnadatta. Her final quarterly report from there, dated 14th August 1915, reads: "6 inpatients, 55 outpatients, 15 tooth extractions, 11 Sabbath evening services, 20 Sunday School sessions, 1 funeral service."

She describes her exit in September 1915 in a buggy along with a young wife going up North to join her husband:

> My companion climbed up to the seat beside the driver, while I clambered up behind and perched sideways, high on top of the luggage and bedding.
> Half the village was out to see us start off, and amidst shouts of farewell and warnings that I should be "back in three weeks", we plunged forward, rattling over the stones, and in a short time were leaving the village behind us, while our lively horses carried us forward into the—to us—unknown.

The horses were certainly lively, and displayed a mind of their own. At one point the driver had to make a rush down a creek bank if they were to have any hope of making it up the other side. Jean remained perched on top of the luggage during the attempt:

> We were almost at the bottom of the incline when the horses in the lead stopped dead, and the speed of the pole horses

and weight of the buggy sent the pole in amongst the leaders' legs. The leaders jumped out of the traces and went back up the hill, taking the pole horses around with them; they being controlled by nothing but the tangled reins, the driver having been thrown out on to his head at the first bump.

Somehow, through all this, Jean retained her precarious perch on top of the luggage. The lead horses stopped eventually and soon they were all on the road again. However, the bumping, swaying and jolting of the coach left them as shaky as jelly by the evening.

Their coachman was a well-known bachelor who came in for some good-natured ribbing from his mates along the way, and gave delight to the Aborigines who believed he had got himself two wives.

Jean liked the young bride with whom she travelled but feared for her future happiness. Typically haughty, she expressed this to Flynn:

> She is a very bright and a good girl but all the people say he [her husband] is a livery individual and do not think much of her chances of enjoying things out there. I wonder more and more how these girls can choose money rather than better things.

After a number of adventures and a long, arduous journey of nine days, Jean arrived at last in Alice Springs. At that time it comprised only around fifty whites and Chinese and their families, but there were also several hundred Aborigines living in nearby camps and many people of all races in the surrounding cattle and mining industries. The town itself disappointed her:

> On the left one passes a well and troughs for watering stock; then an Aboriginal camp and their starving dogs, and on the north side is another camp. And in the midst of all lies the little white settlement, made up of two private houses, two stores, a hotel, policeman's houses, Chinese and Afghans' houses and two corrugated iron sheds for the half-caste children.

However, her welcome was warm and Ida showed her around. Ida's "school" was run in a cramped little stone building behind the main police station. It became the unmarried Constables' quarters later on. Still within the police compound, the "Bungalow" was the sarcastic name given to the iron sheds in which lived the mixed-race children to whom Ida was now "Matron".

Ida explained: "Topsy Smith was living with a white miner in Arltunga, and when he died she brought their five half-caste children here to Sergeant Stott. She was destitute and also wanted protection for her family. He didn't know what to do, so put up a tent for them and contacted Darwin. The Administrator agreed to these iron sheds being built for them, and other half-castes, on the police grounds. Stott looked after them to begin with, but I was offered to be matron and accepted. Topsy is my house-parent and does a fine job, I might add. She teaches the older ones home duties, including sewing, in the mornings while I am teaching the white children. Then in the afternoon I teach fourteen of the half-caste children for an hour and a half, and some of them are showing great promise. It's all an experiment, nothing like it has been done before."

"But that corrugated iron can't supply much shelter. Surely it is too hot during the day and too cold at night?"

"Yes, you're right. I have asked for better accommodation but it will probably be a long time coming. The cooking and bathing facilities are also inadequate, but it is a lot better than most unprotected half-castes are experiencing in the North. What I would like is a hostel out of town. Already Stott has had to shoo away some white men who are eyeing the half-caste girls. He also keeps away tribal and camp blacks other than the mothers. We are hoping to prove that the half-caste can enter white society if given a proper chance. And this year I have a boy of Chinese and Aboriginal descent, who is taught alongside the whites in the mornings, who has actually topped the school in all-round performance. I'm delighted."

Jean met Topsy, a sombre dark-eyed woman in her forties, and looked over the little compound. It was unfenced, unclean, opposite the prison door and too close for comfort to the pub. She found it depressing but did not say so to Ida.

Jean and Ida shared the same large room.

Within a short time, Jean became aware that there were problems between Ida and Sergeant Stott. It transpired that Ida had been seeing a Mr Baker, a married man whom Stott disliked intensely and had ordered not to come to his home. Ida was strong-willed and there were arguments. Jean, always critical, wrote to Flynn:

> I am alarmed at the state of things; she is utterly changed from what she seemed when I saw her in Oodnadatta. She seems to be completely under the influence of that man, yet she knows fully what he is and that his condition of ill health is the result of his awful life. They are on the most familiar terms... Everyone is talking of it but it makes no impression on her. Her husband is still living and it is reported that his [Baker's] wife is living. He had to be ordered away by Stott and now Mrs Standley is always over there. She is a good woman yet so completely influenced by his stronger will. She says: "If my friendship will help him to be better, I will stick to him and the more that people talk the more I shall go to him."

Jean, wisely, stayed out of the conflict between Ida and Robert Stott that had worsened gradually. She wanted to escape to a place of her own, but there was no accommodation available. She asked the pioneer and jack-of-all-trades Sam Nicker to help. He lived in the town and had been one of those who had encouraged her to come in the first place, assuring her that accommodation would be no problem. He looked embarrassed and said he would see what he could do.

She threw herself into her work. Within a few weeks she wrote:

> Since my arrival I have treated cardiac dropsy, fracture of the arm, midwifery case, septic leg, septic hand, lacerated hand, rheumatism, injury to foot, inflamed eyes, injury to back, spider bite, disorder of nerves, gastric disorder of children, extraction of teeth, venereal disease in all its forms.

There could be no lingering doubt about the need for medical services to be supplied to Alice Springs. Flynn wrote happily in the *Inlander* at the close of 1915:

> It is now easier for families to go back there. One man hesitated a long time about bringing his family all the way from Sydney, but at last he did so – before either teacher or nurse had actually arrived. Then he nearly decided to send them away again, but the advent of teacher and nurse have altered the position.

Remembering Flynn's goal of encouraging more women to live in the outback, we can understand his enthusiasm.

With no room to act as a dispensary or clinic, Jean spent as much time as she could nursing the sick in their own homes. She had a radius of 240 kilometres to cover and so spent much time on gruelling visits to cattle stations outside the town, helping the sick when and where she could. The countryside was in the grip of a terrible drought. "The stench of dying stock is in your nostrils most places you go, but especially around the dry water holes and bores. The flies are overwhelming and I wear a net".

Partly because of her choice to distance herself from the Stotts ("splendid people") and from Ida, Jean found life busy but lonely:

> In my lonely wanderings I visited the local burial place, where I found evidence of the many who had passed by that way and had fallen. I waylaid Aboriginal women and tried to know them better. I wandered about the hills enjoying the solitude, at times accompanied by newly made [Aboriginal] friends.

Her fondness for Aborigines was shared by many of the AIM nurses who followed her. One expressed it in these sentiments: "To us from the cities, they appeared strange, but as we came to know and appreciate their friendliness and helpfulness we accepted them gladly into the AIM family."

Jean's growing companionship with Aborigines increased when she was spooked by a cow:

> Now, I never care to meet with a strange cow in any part of the country unless there is also a fence handy – there is no fence in Central Australia. This cow looked at me with suspicion, turned around and pranced, turned again and

pranced, put down her head and watched me. I gathered together my skirt and made one wild, terrified rush right into the midst of the Aboriginal camp... They waved their arms above their heads and rocked and rolled with laughter.

I was indignant at such untimely mirth and said, "I have been frightened by that cow."

When they could control their mirth sufficiently to be able to speak, they gasped out, "That cow been frighten longa you."

Then one dusky girl came to my aid. "You frighten? Me go longa you."

She proceeded to accompany me. When I reached the telegraph station, and was parting from my escort, I handed her some pennies.

On the return journey, a couple of hours later, half the female portion of the camp were out waiting to accompany me home again. There were no more pennies but a few sweets did just as well.

Ever after this I never went out without a supply of sweets. For never after this did I lack an escort whatever direction I might take. And those simple women saw to it that some harmless little calf, or half-starved cow, was somewhere in my path, as an excuse for their offer to accompany me. However, I was grateful for their simple act of friendliness.

The Aborigines, especially a woman named Triff, thereby helped to ease Jean's loneliness. One day Triff curled down on a stone beside where Jean sat on a boulder and put her hand gently on Jean's shoulder. "Poor Nussa all alone; that no good. One fella all alone; that no good." Jean was touched by her show of concern and commented, "She had touched on part of the problem of a nurse in the Centre—'one fella all alone, no good'."

Jean had been sent to uncover problems, so she wrote to Flynn to say that nurses must serve with companions or in pairs to ease the loneliness.

The second major problem, unsuitable accommodation, grew worse not better. But when Jean had to run a clinic or treat an infectious case, the obliging Sergeant Stott would occasionally clear the jail for her to use. This was not the first time it had been used for unusual activity; Jessie Litchfield records in her (unpublished) *Historical Review of the Northern Territory*:

> When Sir Thomas Bridges was Governor of South Australia, he came to Alice Springs with Sir Henry Barwell. A dance was held in the lock-up: the prisoners were taken out of it, the whole place was cleaned and decorated, and the chains on the wall were covered with greenery.

The police buildings were also used for Sunday School and Services, but were inadequate. These were held in the little room where Ida taught school, the "Prison Warder's Room". Jean gamely took weekly church services until "the weather became too hot for the people to be in a small room, even for a short time, and the ravings of a mad black man in the prison next door when he heard our voices was too terrible to endure".

The discord in the Stotts' house widened, as is so often the case. The fact that Stott had the responsibility to oversee Ida's work was not a comfortable arrangement. "She is not a good manager and is rather overworked with the school and he is a born bully who wants to interfere. Things are desperately unsettled," Jean noted anxiously.

In fact, they became so unsettled that Jean could no longer trust herself not to say something. She decided she had to find somewhere else to stay no matter how unsuitable. Sam Nicker and others finally acted on her behalf, choosing a deserted room, once used as a shop, beside a slab hut named "Myrtle Villa".

> The only available building was the square shell of an old shop, which some old bushmen undertook to put in order for me. They cleared out the cellar, mended the roof [in part only] and put up a tent in the middle of it; then made table, deck chair and all that they could think of for comfort so that I had a room quite to myself except for the friendly lizards, which sported about the walls... About a hundred yards from my little home was a stony hill, from which, I was assured, "snakes always come at this time of the year" and was told I must "be careful never to go about at night without a lantern"; and to search my tent "and

never put your foot on the floor till you have made a light".
I determined to follow all the instructions most carefully.

The time had come to take her leave of the Stotts. In January 1916 she described to Flynn her leaving:

> I departed from the Stotts house last week, in order to be near Mrs Hayes during her illness, the excuse is good enough. I have gone nearly mad trying to keep out of old Stott's and Mrs Standley's brawls, which come thick and fast. I thanked Mr and Mrs Stott for what they had done, but I had reached the last straw on the lines of peace. [She then described her tent in the old shop and swore Flynn to secrecy.] Don't you tell anyone because I could never make my sister understand that I am quite safe.

A major problem with the old shop was that it had no doors. Early mornings young children would chase the goats into it for milking, waking her up in her tent. Also it was used as a thoroughfare while she was attending to patients and the number of whites calling on her services dwindled. Her inability to gain the friendship and support of some key whites also resulted in fewer whites seeking her aid in proportion to the Aborigines who came. She expressed this frustration in her recommendations of March 1915:

> A medical missionary will be of greater service here than a nurse. The postmaster and policeman are in the habit of being unofficial doctors so they interfere and a man may be able to help them more. Of course, working like this, a nurse is not employed in the ordinary way; if she were, I should have no difficulty in dealing with interference.

She explained further that, being a woman, she did not feel she could tell men that they had venereal diseases as that would cause trouble. A male doctor could do so.

Soon afterwards, the Nicker family moved out of their old slab cabin, Myrtle Villa, to develop a station "up the track". Their buggy actually broke down irreparably at Ryan's Well, where they established a new homestead and station quite successfully. But on their leaving Alice Springs, Jean moved at once into Myrtle Villa and it became known as "Sister's Hospital":

> My slab cabin had two small rooms with a kitchen a few yards away. My room had a fireplace. The ceiling of calico was full of gaping wounds… the whole interior was black with smoke. My black assistant [Maude], who was big and strong, occupied the next room. Each night we placed our bunks out under the sky, one on each side of the door. As I peered about and asked, "Do you think there are any snakes about?" Maude reassured me, "Don't you bin frighten, Nussa. I not let anytings hurt you. I got big stick—kill 'em." Any late visitor would have met with a lively reception.

Maude was also there with Jean during a frightening dust storm:

> We see to the south, swirling high above the mountain range, one huge wall of brown sand—miles of it—the whole length of the range as far as the eye could see. Dogs go into hiding; horses and camels tremble and become restless. We shut doors and windows and go into the stifling heat of the house. It is upon us at last, and in spite of doors and windows the dust pours in. I cover my head with a pillowcase and wait, feeling that the house must be swept away. Hour after hour through the night it rages. I beat my hands on the partition dividing our room, and beg Maude not to go to sleep, for I feel that I shall not be able to breathe much longer. But the sound of even breathing tells me that the storm is not keeping Maude awake! In time it has spent its fury and subsides.

That was Maude's main weakness as a "protector"; she could sleep through "anyting".

Jean's isolation accentuated her loneliness. She lamented: "I have experienced what it is like to be utterly alone, without any means of escaping from the isolation."

Her mother became seriously ill and Jean asked to leave her post a month early, to be with her. She had fulfilled her mission in that she could give first-hand advice to Flynn. Her final analysis was that more than just a nurse was needed, but that a doctor and a dust-proof hospital were both required. "Call it a hospital, and charge for everything". She added that a clubroom for healthy social activities should also be considered by the AIM.

Jean gamely rode a lively horse on her return. After a number of days they reached the railhead at Oodnadatta. Then she returned home to Melbourne by train to nurse her mother.

There are many levels on which to evaluate Jean's contribution. Through no fault of her own, her effectiveness was dogged by unsatisfactory relationships with some of the powerful whites in the region. Perhaps her friendship with Aborigines had a part to play in her marginalisation by certain racial elements in the community, and she criticised these attitudes in an article in 1937 in the Messenger. But was her critical nature partly to blame for some of the discord and rejection? She herself told Flynn: "A silly old matron once said that I was the easiest kind of person to fall out with", and perhaps that matron's analysis was accurate. For example, she became very critical of the great Bruce Plowman, and he of her. He, though, was extraordinarily popular in the region and she was not. Later on, he even wrote to the church magazine, the *Messenger*, complaining that she had done the AIM harm by rejecting some local offers of land. Jean replied that the land in question had been offered in gratitude after she had saved a child's life and that it would have been inappropriate to accept it. Furthermore, "as it was near the hotel and beside the house of an Afghan and Chinese drinking shop, it was useless as a site for a hostel".

Years later Jean Whitla, Plowman's daughter, returned to her father's old haunts. She was treated like family and regaled with stories about how wonderfully Bruce had served in the Centre. She also found some elderly pioneers who remembered Jean Finlayson and spoke highly of her nursing achievements, but said she had not been well-liked on a personal level.

Beyond personal issues, her nursing service was agreed by one and all to be quite outstanding. A grateful Alice Springs has named Finlayson Street and Finlayson Park in her honour.

On what passions was Jean's sacrificial service based? We turn to her writings and find a deep empathy with everyone who suffered. We discover her as a lonely white figure in the local graveyard, which she visited a number of times, sobbing aloud as she reads the gravestones. She wrote for the *Messenger* in February 1916:

> There is a graveyard in the midst of which stand two solitary ironbark trees, through which the wind moans and forces one to feel a greater sadness when visiting this spot… One neat little stone bears the name of a brave young woman who came with her husband into the midst of a desert to share his dangers and rough, lonely life. What she suffered in isolation from other women, only a bush-woman of similar experience could understand. Suffering from fever, she died, leaving a tiny baby girl. On one stone is inscribed the name of a young man of 22 years, and underneath it the words, "In the midst of Life we are in Death"… As the wind moans through these two old ironbark trees, one weeps for the human suffering that has been.

Jean had one final contribution to make to Central Australia; John Flynn sought her advice when designing a cottage hospital for Alice Springs. Jean was adamant that cool, clean air was important to the healing process and Flynn decided on a unique design that cooled all air by drawing it through an underground tunnel past wet sacking. She also recommended verandahs wide enough to put beds out on summer nights and many other practical features. Flynn completed the hospital, named Adelaide House, in 1926. How different Jean's year would have been if Flynn's hospital had been there for her. But it had been crafted in the anvil of her tough experiences, and from that she could draw satisfaction.

What happened to the major players in the Inland with whom Jean had overlapped?

Sister Latto Bett served with distinction during the First World War. She married one of the servicemen whom she nursed and they returned to Australia to live. Popular and respected, she spoke highly of Flynn and defended allegations of racism against the AIM in 1937. She was surprised but delighted to be honoured by a brass plaque in her name at the John Flynn Church in Alice Springs in 1956.

Sergeant Robert Stott was promoted to Commissioner Stott and became a legend. He was sometimes, though not always kindly, referred to as "the uncrowned king of Alice Springs" because he supplied strong leadership in an otherwise leaderless community. Mount Stott and Stott Terrace in Alice Springs are named after him.

Ida Standley, later Dame Ida Standley, moved into Myrtle Villa as soon as Jean had vacated it. The Bungalow had been built to house twelve only, but by 1927 it was hopelessly overcrowded and many of the seventy children slept in the yard. Indeed, when it rained, there was not enough room indoors for all to crowd in. This encouraged further the sexual problems Jean had foreseen with the pub so close by. Dr Walker described the pitiful situation in a report he wrote for the Government:

> It is situated within 30 yards of the rear entrance to the hotel and is a direct invitation to men under the influence of liquor. The female half-castes are nothing but "public property". I am told that to go near at night and whistle is all that is necessary.

Not unexpectedly, this resulted in a new generation of unwanted illegitimate babies to care for at the Bungalow, the young mothers and babies having nowhere else to go. Ida continued to smile her way through all the traumas and dramas and numbers swelled. Three, four and up to five children of any sex would share the same blanket lying on the floor or in the yard. Ida still provided a rudimentary education for all her charges and supervised the meals, bread-making, laundry and sewing. Several visitors remarked on the cleanliness of the children and their clothing as a credit to her.

It took until 1929 before the Bungalow was moved to Jay Creek, but the accommodation was almost as poor—Ida living in a tent inside a bough shelter and the children inside a tin shed constructed using material from the original Bungalow. At least her charges were now separated from the drunken men at the hotel.

Ida remained a staunch supporter of Flynn and the AIM and served for years on the committee that raised funds for an AIM hospital. She had become part of that wider support for his vision that he always courted, believing that all women should network into a caring community in the bush. Flynn referred to Ida in his 1927 *Inlander* article as "Ma'" and later as "Beloved Lady". Her health finally broke down in 1929 when she was aged sixty. That same year she was awarded the MBE for her service to child welfare and later Standley Chasm and various streets and a school were named after her in Alice Springs. Perhaps her greatest success was the scholastic achievements of her pupils, against the odds, which caused whites to see part-Aborigines in a new and more favourable light.

And Myrtle Villa? All traces of it have long since disappeared. A daughter of Ida Standley in 1987 unveiled a plaque where it once stood. There is now a petrol station at the site.

Minnie Kinnear at Innamincka

After Jean Finlayson's harrowing experiences of nursing without proper accommodation, Flynn determined never to repeat the experiment. However, the men and women of the Channel country heard how successfully Jean had served and approached Flynn to provide them with a single nurse 'like Sister Bett or Sister Finlayson' to serve at Innamincka. Flynn was involved in other nursing ventures that stretched his resources and he had to demur for the time being.

Flynn established new AIM hospitals and nurses for Port Hedland, Maranboy, Beltana and Hall's Creek. The years slipped by but the needs of 'Tragedy Corner', where Queensland, New South Wales and South Australia shared common borders, kept impinging themselves on him through accounts of great suffering there.

He communicated with the managers of the four largest cattle properties in the Channel Country: Innamincka, Cordillo Downs, Nappa Merrie and Arrabury. Each had a considerable workforce; for example there were around 150 whites on Cordillo Downs and fifty on Arrabury. He informed them he would consider putting an itinerant nurse there to serve the community, rather like his Patrol Padres did. However, drawing on Jean's difficulties, he explained he would not do so unless she was assured of good accommodation at one or more of the homesteads. Based on these discussions, the managers of the four largest cattle stations met in 1923 to formalise a proposal to put to Flynn: that they would host the Border Nurse in turn. She would hold clinics first on one property, then the next, and so on unless medical needs dictated she went elsewhere. Each property would supply her with a room and board and also provide somewhere suitable for her to examine patients. They even offered to pay her salary. Though uneasy about it, Flynn agreed to the Border Nurse concept, though he did not assume full responsibility for it in the beginning.

Who should Flynn recommend for this "boundary-riding" nurse? Drawing on Jean's example, he decided she must be a nurse who was already serving with success in the bush and had shown a high degree of adaptability and initiative, for example in making diagnoses and undertaking medical treatment without communicating with a doctor. The nearest doctor to Innamincka would be hundreds of miles away across forbidding territory. She would need to be on duty every day for 24 hours and be capable of conducting burial services, delivering babies and counselling disturbed men or women. Regarding personal comforts, she must be able to survive the hottest of weather, camp under the stars, drink brackish bore water and eat dried salt beef and damper only for days on end. Most importantly, she must be able to ride a horse or camel over long, drought-affected distances. These requirements were very limiting. Indeed, only one candidate really fulfilled them. Her name was Marjorie Kinnear, more commonly known as Minnie.

Flynn held Minnie in high regard. As early as January 1919 he had written to Nell Inglis and described Minnie as "the sort that will play the game in any corner you put her, even if she is an 'Anglican'!... I think she is a good sport and with a true soul".

Within four years the corner in which he would ask her to "play the game" would be the fearsome "Tragedy Corner", where explorers Burke and Wills had perished.

Before then, Minnie had the honour of being the first Sister-in-Charge of Flynn's new cottage hospital, "The Mitchell Home", in Beltana. She had a companion there in Miss Jean MacLeod to help with the cooking and menial tasks, but not with the nursing. Minnie had set high standards for the hospital and Flynn was delighted with her efforts because, as he explained to her: "A thing

75

done well becomes a tradition that those who come after must live up to."

But could she or any other nurse take on successfully the awesome task of Innamincka? The one cattle property, that of Innamincka itself, leased by the "Cattle King" Sir Sidney Kidman, covered 11,000 square miles. When the other cattle properties and associated areas were added, her "field" stretched across an area that was half the size of Victoria, for which she would have direct responsibility. For a woman who had lived and trained in Victoria, that concept was daunting. Worse still, she discovered she would have no access to telephone, wireless or telegraph over that whole vast region. Messages would have to be carried by horse, foot, camel, motor or word-of-mouth, the last technique being known locally as the "mulga wire".

Minnie found out all she could about the region.

The explorer Charles Sturt was in 1845 the first Europen to see the region. He had named Cooper Creek and found a vast gibber plain now named Sturt's Stony Desert. What photographs Minnie could find showed cloudless skies and rocks stretching to the horizon. Not an easy landscape over which to ride or take a motor.

Sturt's explorations had been followed in 1860 by the Burke and Wills expedition, which had built a depot at Innamincka. On their return, Burke and Wills both died there within a few miles of the present township. Carvings on trees and gravesites showed where the tragedy had occurred. In 1870 John Conrick drove a mob of cattle there and took up land locally. Other settlers soon followed him. By 1923 the township of Innamincka had grown to service the local region and also the drovers who crossed the Cooper nearby. Minnie found out that it comprised a police station, hotel, a store and a couple of shabby iron houses. The hotel was gaining renown for its pile of empty discarded bottles, a pile that was destined to grow to 200 metres long by 2 high and 7 wide, and "the biggest in the world".

It was into this thirsty, incredibly hot, dry and forbidding region that Minnie was posted, to act alone without medical support of any sort.

Not wishing to repeat the weaknesses discovered during the Jean Finlayson experiment, Flynn asked his good friend and Medical Advisor, Dr George Simpson, to vet the task in advance.

Simpson visited the region and was struck by the desolation. He advised each cattle station how to set up a room as an "Outpatients Clinic" for Minnie.

On his return to the city, Simpson helped Minnie to equip each homestead with bulk medicines, surgical instruments and a variety of drugs. The lines of transport were long and replacing stocks would take three months, so careful planning was vital.

In 1923 she was ready and was sent out to pioneer the Border Nurse experiment. A tiny woman in her early thirties, slim and dark-haired, she hardly looked adequate to the challenges that lay ahead. Her small stature belied the steely resolve with which she approached the overwhelming task.

She walked right into a deadly influenza epidemic! She reported that every morning fresh victims were brought to her attention. She rode around to the sufferers, who were often lying in shearing sheds, rough huts, or even on the ground under inadequate shade in the stockyard. She would dismount, take temperatures, apply compresses and dispense medicine. If she could, she would remain with the man until the crisis had passed. Fred Debney, the manager of Arrabury station, stated later, "I don't know what we would have done without Sister Kinnear during the epidemic. She worked day and night to save lives."

The epidemic eased, but she was always busy.

> There were midnight journeys over rough bush tracks to a sudden call and camps out in the bush on the way.

Besides the local stockmen, station-hands, shearers and managers, she treated itinerant Aborigines, Afghan cameleers, swagmen, rouseabouts and the drovers who used the Strzelecki Track. In September she listed the variety of cases she had treated in the preceding few weeks, among them "retention of urine, sandy blight, food poisoning, tooth extractions, infected arm, broken bones, scurvy, influenza, pain in the side, confinement and septicaemia". And things had quietened down somewhat by then.

Broken bones were set without the benefit of X-rays. Septicaemia and infections of the eyes were treated with mild antiseptics because antibiotics had not yet been discovered.

However, a nurse could not treat certain medical conditions. Such cases, often urgent, required a doctor. There were no roads in the region, only rough tracks. The pain and trauma suffered by those who were bounced around for days to reach a doctor could only be imagined. One family had to take their baby to a doctor 500 kilometres away. They motored gamely all afternoon and into the night, but the baby's condition worsened. At 1 a.m. she died. A camping sheet was spread on the ground beside the deserted track and the man walked back a distance to fetch water to prepare her little body for burial. Then the parents had to continue their journey in order to obtain an official Order For Burial. Another young man was diagnosed by Minnie with acute appendicitis and had to be driven 320 kilometres to the doctor at Tibooburra. Operated on immediately he arrived, his life was saved, but only after hours of throbbing pain.

Many times she had to accompany those who were dangerously sick on a cattle train:

> One was a boy, terribly ill. We travelled all night, and as soon as the jolting of the train began he became delirious. I had to get the cattle men to help me keep him in the carriage.

This boy pulled through eventually and another life was saved.

But a man was brought to her suffering from dreadful internal injuries after being kicked and trodden on by a horse. He begged her not to send him to the hospital because he could not face the agonies that he would have to suffer just to get there. She was nonplussed and decided to treat him herself. He appeared to respond well to the treatment she gave him, but took a turn for the worse during a heat wave with the temperature at 50°C in the shade. Minnie decided he needed an operation to survive. Once again, the man begged her not to send him away. She could not telephone or telegraph for advice, the nearest telegraph being 600 kilometres away. He would have to be sent for an operation to the nearest hospital at Port Augusta. This would involve being thrown about in a buggy while travelling over rough tracks for 640 kilometres, and then being put on a train for a further 320 kilometres. Oh, why was Flynn's dream of a Flying Doctor taking so long? Always a vocal supporter of his vision of a Mantle of Safety, at that moment she saw how it could make the difference between life and death for her patient.

Professionally speaking, despite his protests, she had no choice:

> It was a forlorn hope that the patient would survive the terrible journey in mid-summer, but as it was the only hope, preparations were made. Before we could set out, the patient died, and I was glad that he was spared the long agony of travelling over the rough sand-hills and stony plains.

Her services to the dead man were not yet over because she had to organise his burial. She arranged with the local policeman to make a coffin. (His coffins were roughly hewn. He had to make a number of them that year.) Then she conducted the burial service itself.

Minnie found it necessary to improvise during a number of emergencies. For example, when faced with the fracture of a stockman's leg caused by falling off a horse, Minnie had nothing with her from which to make a splint. Casting around desperately, she took a thin, crooked branch off a tree. With careful bandaging firmer than usual, she managed to get the patient back to Cordillo Downs successfully.

For the men and women of that vast region, it was a great relief to have a nurse in the vicinity:

> All round the three stations, and from beyond them, came calls from people who had been nursing their own in anxiety and fearful strain. Most of them had never seen a trained nurse's uniform before, but they were pathetically eager for help and advice. The cases were hundreds of miles apart, all separated by rough bush tracks.

Minnie overflowed with praise for the kindliness and courtesy she was shown.

> I nursed a man with double pneumonia once in a little harness shed, and the only fire we had was made of sticks

poked through the top of an oil drum. The cook's off-sider used to come along after the night duty with hot tea and toast. How kind they were, all the bush people! I have never known in the roughest shearing shed the slightest discourtesy to any woman. Always for the suffering, there was the greatest kindness and care. It was a fascinating life and I loved it.

Minnie gives us a picture of the women on stations at that time and the hardships they faced:

> There are few white women there—only the station managers' wives, with one married couple on nearly every station and no other women within hundreds of miles. The women who do go up there are magnificent. They have a courage we can hardly imagine. Year after year—one woman has been there for twenty—they stand shoulder to shoulder with their husbands, never complaining, always cheerful. They may not notice it, but they grow old quickly. Childbirth means such weary journeys, such loneliness, such anxiety as no city woman can ever imagine. And their children may fall ill and die without ever a doctor or nurse at call... And bush babies, remember, are just as precious and lovable as city babies.

Conditions were hard on her also. The diet was inadequate. The sandflies were terrible and even crawled under the sheets at night to bite. On one occasion, she saw several dogs standing downwind in the smoke of a campfire to escape sandflies. On another, she rode 160 kilometres through drought conditions under a burning sun to attend to an emergency call. And then when she arrived she needed to feed the patient something to sustain him, but there was no food available other than salt beef, "no milk because the milking goat had run dry, no fruit or vegetables or butter. All that was suitable was jelly, which had to be made after sundown and put into a tin billy and hung into the water of the well for it to set". And it was too hot to sleep properly in the iron houses in which the temperature rose to 50°C. Even the children would get up in the night to shower to cool down and parents would sprinkle their bedding with water.

Similarly to Jean Finlayson, Minnie had to leave her post before her year was quite completed. In her case her health finally collapsed under the incredible strain. However, she and the people of the Channel Country advised Flynn that the work needed to go on. Flynn decided that a younger nurse might handle the extreme conditions better and that things would be much easier now that Sister Kinnear had pioneered the field. Subsequently, the younger Sister Aleida Levick, who had nursed in country hospitals, was proposed to be the next Border Nurse. Flynn wrote of her:

> Sister Levick is one of our family. She is especially trained for work on the field of the Australian Inland Mission. She is a very lovable girl, and capable as well. I am sure that she will be well liked in the Channel Country.

She was, and did a fine job, giving much of the credit to the foundations laid so thoroughly and bravely by Minnie Kinnear.

In the meantime Minnie took several months in Victoria to recover her strength. But she was not finished with her concerns for Tragedy Corner. Invited to speak at an AIM rally in Melbourne, she described her year as a Border Nurse. Certain young trainee nurses sat enthralled and challenged by what they heard. Minnie was passing the flame on to her listeners, and Elizabeth Burchill was one of those trainees. The talk inspired Elizabeth to play her own part at Innamincka and her subsequent book, *Innamincka*, has become a classic description of nursing in the outback.

Minnie did more at that rally than simply describe her own experiences. She suggested solutions to the problems, most especially promoting Flynn's dream of a wireless network and Flying Doctors. But in the short term she proposed a cottage hospital be built and staffed by two AIM nurses, even just a simple building with enclosed verandas and a cooler cane-grass shed attached. Little did she think that she herself would play a major part in enabling her dream to come true.

To her surprise, her story attracted media attention. The *Adelaide Register* printed a detailed account of her experiences complete with a photograph of the corrugated-iron lean-to at the end of a shearing shed that was the closest she came to having a hospital in which to nurse the sick. Like an oven, it had been of little practical use.

Encouraged, Minnie wrote further articles including one in the *Observer* in March 1924: "Will you kindly grant me space in your columns to plead for the erection of a nursing home at Innamincka immediately?" She proceeded to describe some of the tragedies with which she had been involved. She ended with, "Much suffering of patients, much suspense and anxiety of mothers, and lives of strong, sturdy men, and helpless little children will be saved thereby." The editor added that he would be pleased to receive and acknowledge subscriptions for this cause.

Sir Josiah Symon, a prominent citizen of Adelaide who had already told Flynn he was prepared to support an AIM hospital, read her articles. He was moved by them and wrote forthwith to Flynn. His letter offering help was quoted in the press. Here are excerpts:

> In a city rich in hospitals, trained nurses and skilful physicians, we are apt to forget in our more favoured surroundings, not from want of heart but from want of knowledge, what men and women in the "Never-Never" endure in their time of wounds and sickness. To bring kindness and care to the stricken is the first purpose of your mission, but it is, in my opinion, a means of opening up the distant places of Australia and fitting them for settlement with some share of the amenities of civilisation. From both points of view, I know of no nobler work than that of your mission. Sister Kinnear, through the press, has lately made clear in some detail what it is you are doing and its difficulties. I shall be glad, therefore, if you will allow me to offer some help.

The help he offered was £1500 to build a cottage hospital at Innamincka! This would be sufficient for the basic structure—furnishings and so forth would be extra. The new hospital would be called the "Elizabeth Symon Nursing Home" in honour of Sir Josiah's mother.

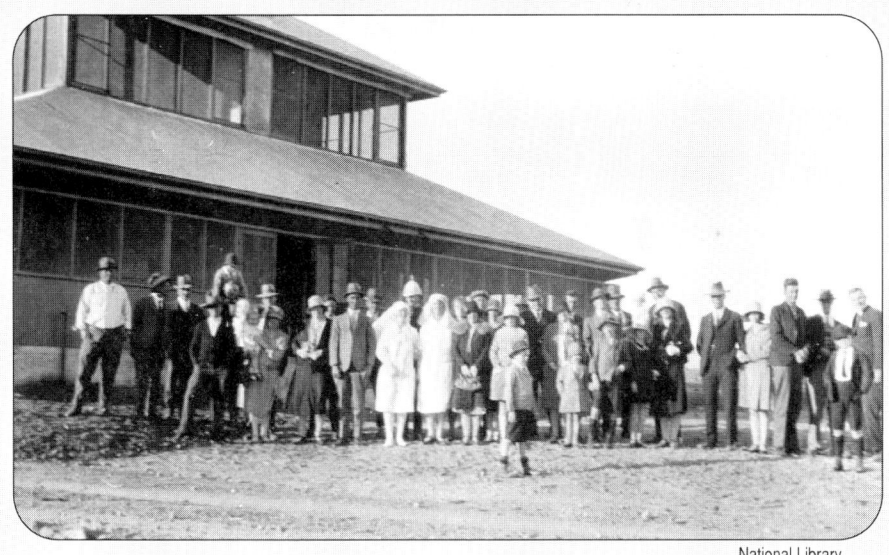

Above: "The finest building in the inland". Opening ceremony for the Elizabeth Symon Nursing Home, Innamincka, in May 1929. The building was designed by Minnie Kinnear and John Flynn. The Nursing Sisters are Claire Stewart and Elspeth Edgar and behind them is the policeman, Jack Ridge. Donning his uniform for the occasion - and for the first time - he attracted hordes of children, who followed him everywhere.

The Elizabeth Symon Nursing Home in 1936. The nurses abandoned the upstairs area during the blistering inland summers, as the corrugated-iron roof turned its rooms into an oven.

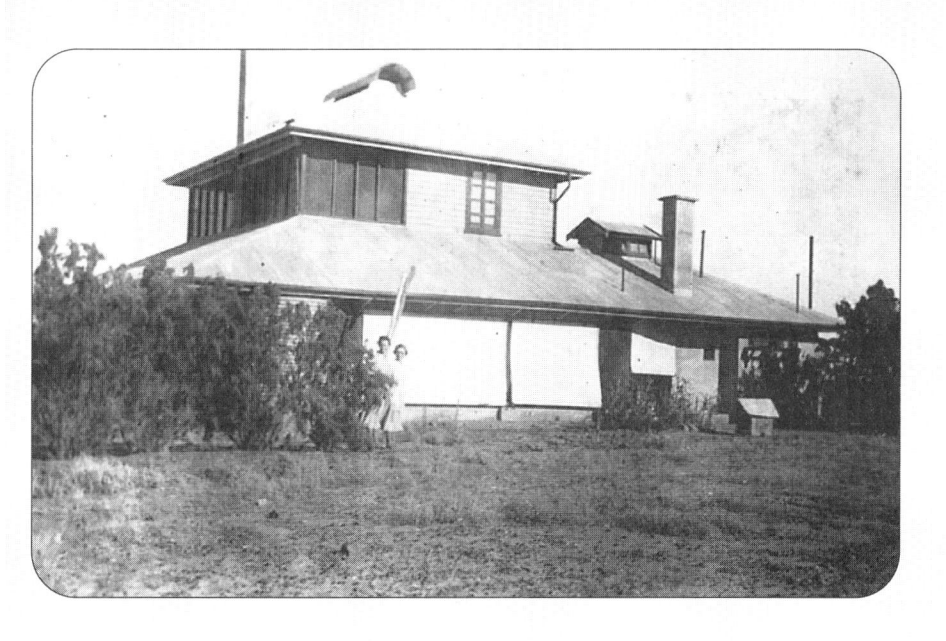

NT Library

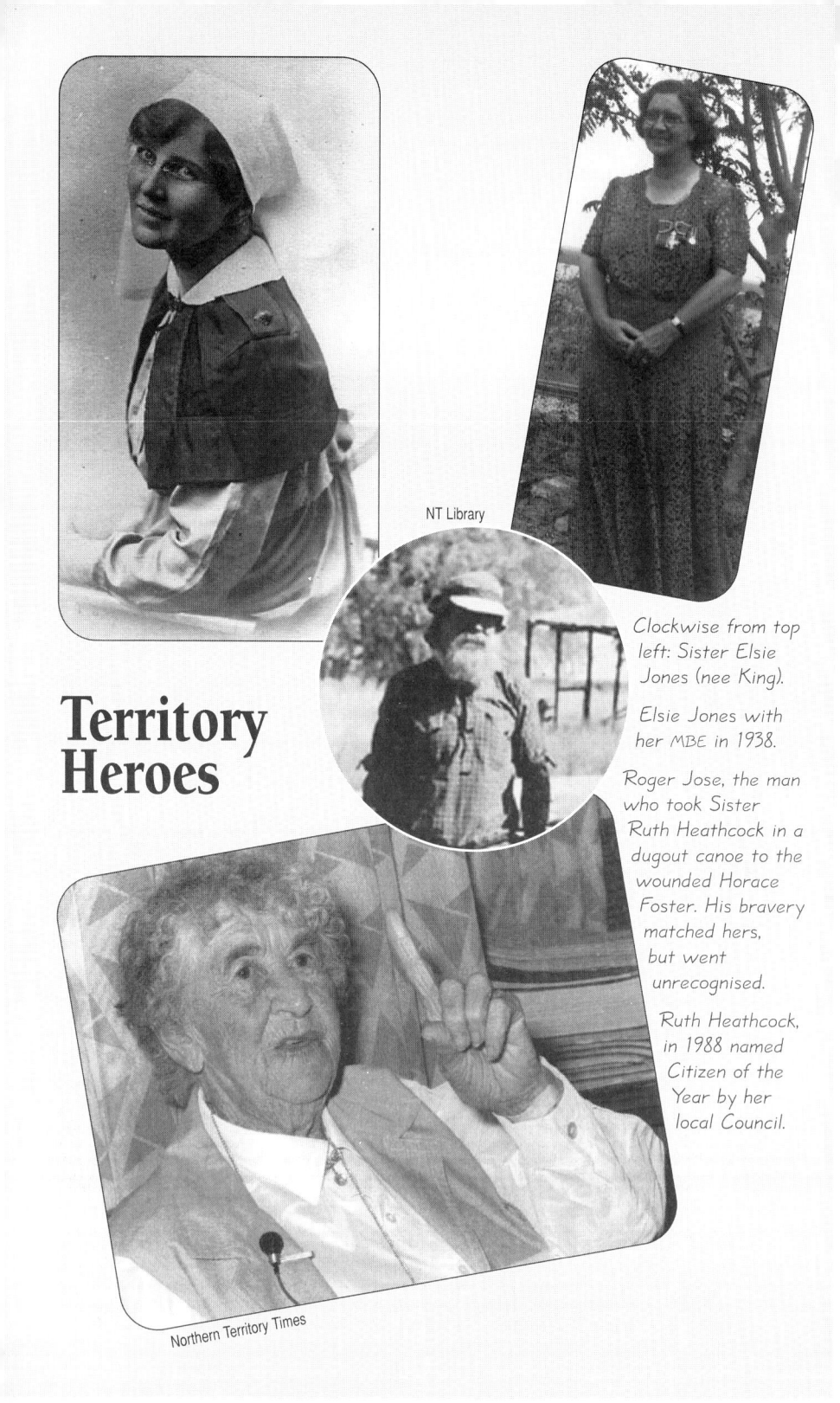

Territory Heroes

Clockwise from top left: Sister Elsie Jones (nee King).

Elsie Jones with her MBE in 1938.

Roger Jose, the man who took Sister Ruth Heathcock in a dugout canoe to the wounded Horace Foster. His bravery matched hers, but went unrecognised.

Ruth Heathcock, in 1988 named Citizen of the Year by her local Council.

Northern Territory Times

Patrol Padres called on the nurses and offered help when they could. Here Fred McKay helps Lillian to carry an injured child to hospital.

Centre: The AIM family provided friendship and support to nurses and locals alike. Here we see Maurie Anderson (wireless expert), Mrs Jean Flynn, Fred McKay, Sisters Alice Anderson and Lillian Cooper and the Ward family at an AIM gathering in Charleville. At the bottom of the page are the Patrol cars in which they travelled.

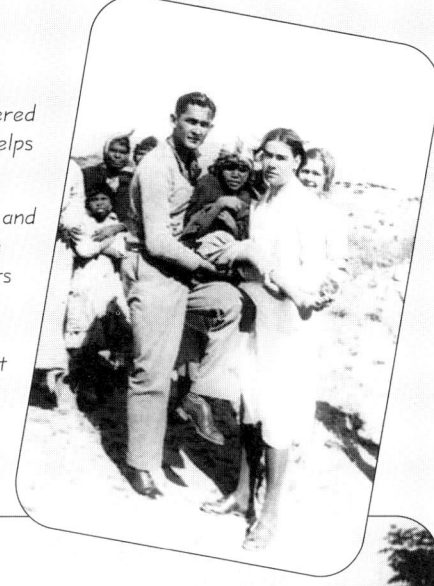

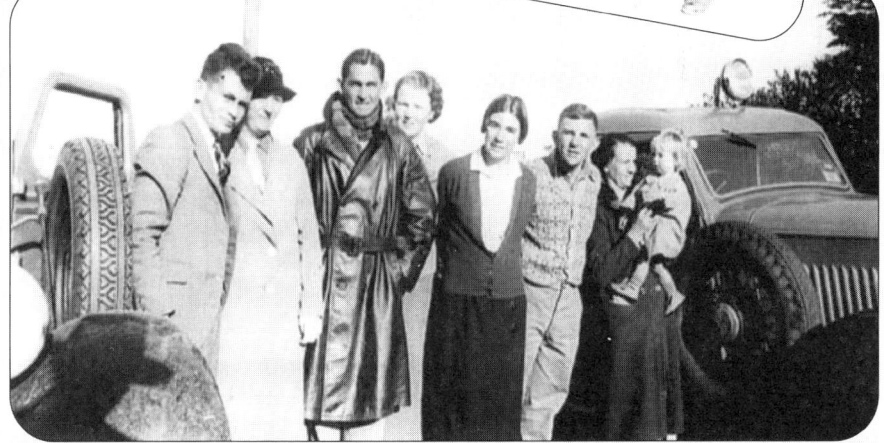

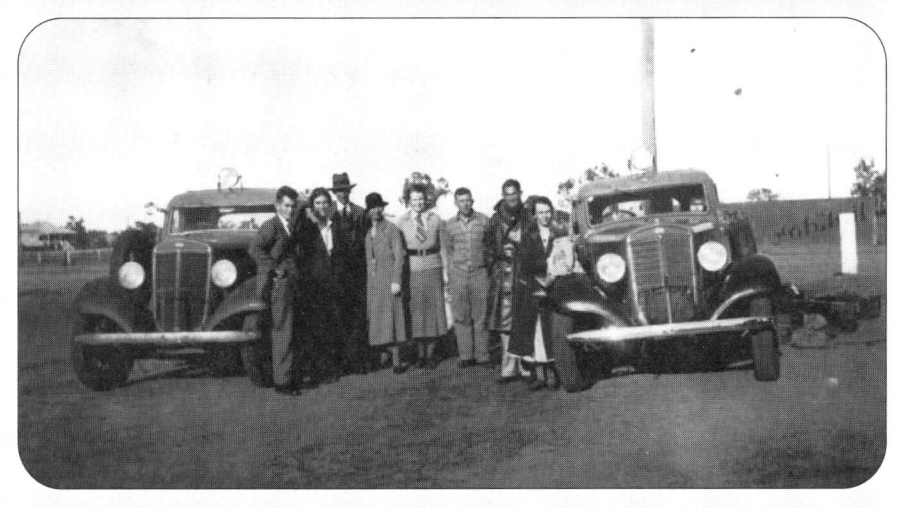

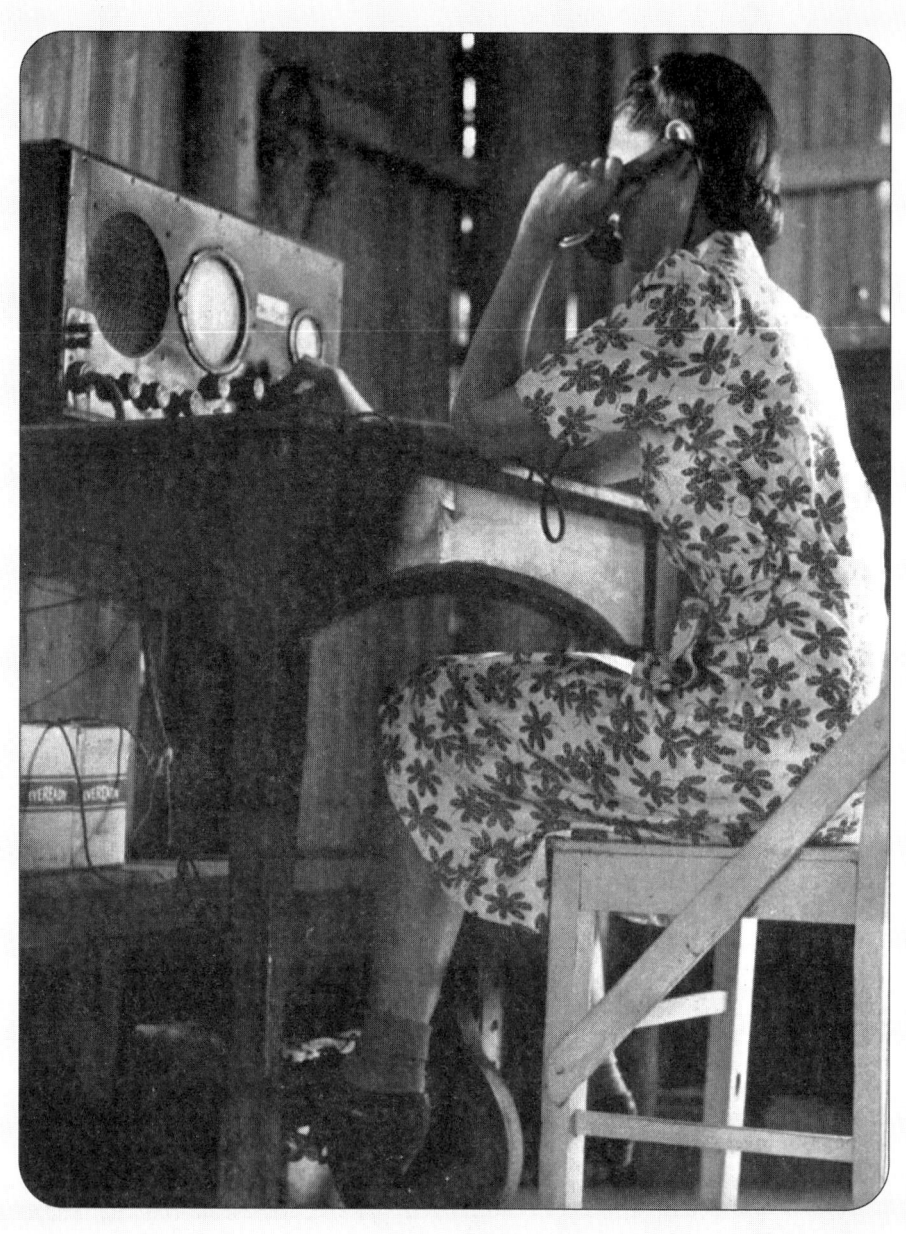

Housewives outback eagerly adopted the new transceiver, using pedal power to chat in "galah sessions", send telegrams and call the Flying Doctor for advice or emergency help.

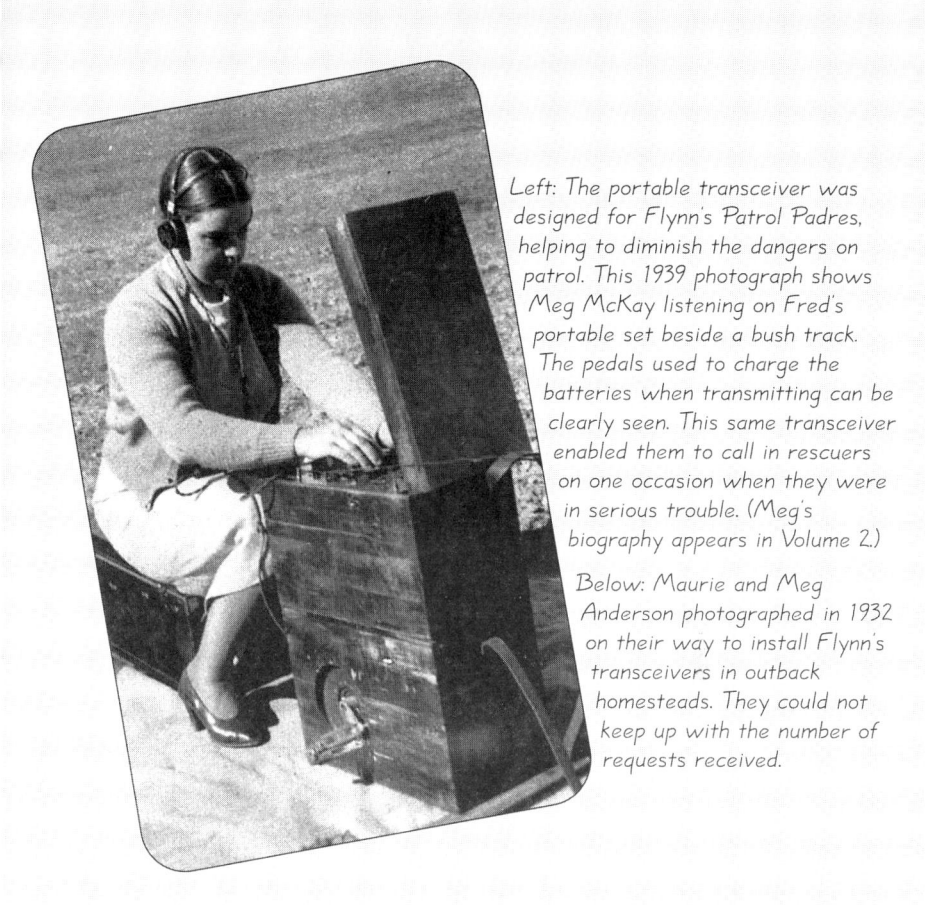

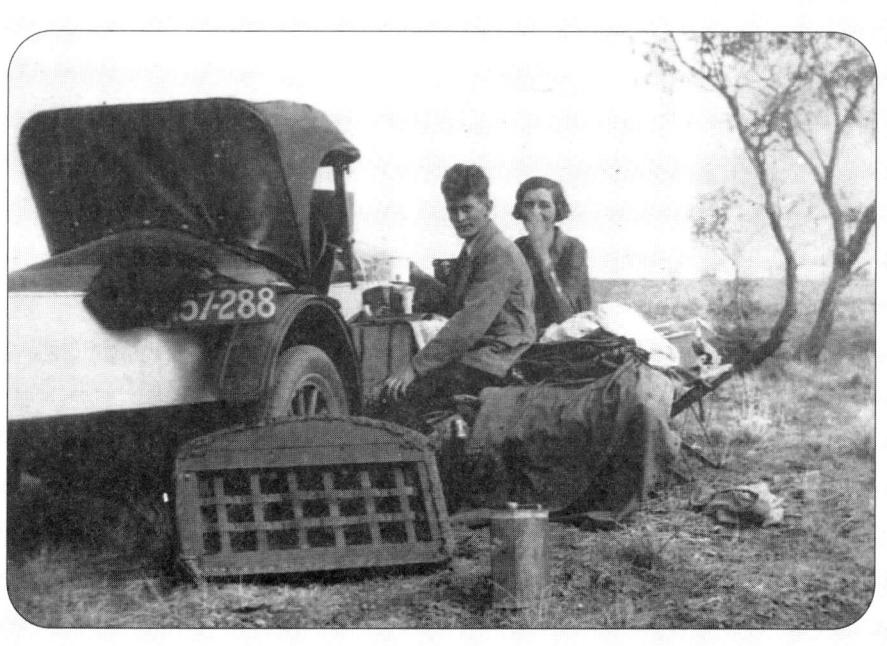

Left: The portable transceiver was designed for Flynn's Patrol Padres, helping to diminish the dangers on patrol. This 1939 photograph shows Meg McKay listening on Fred's portable set beside a bush track. The pedals used to charge the batteries when transmitting can be clearly seen. This same transceiver enabled them to call in rescuers on one occasion when they were in serious trouble. (Meg's biography appears in Volume 2.)

Below: Maurie and Meg Anderson photographed in 1932 on their way to install Flynn's transceivers in outback homesteads. They could not keep up with the number of requests received.

Getting to Birdsville

Patrol Padre Fred McKay transported the new Sisters to Birdsville in 1936. Lillian Cooper and Alice Anderson helped when the truck was bogged in mud and they saw the isolation in which the pioneers lived at lonely outposts like Pandi-Pandi station. At night they camped beside the track until at last they reached their destination - Birdsville.

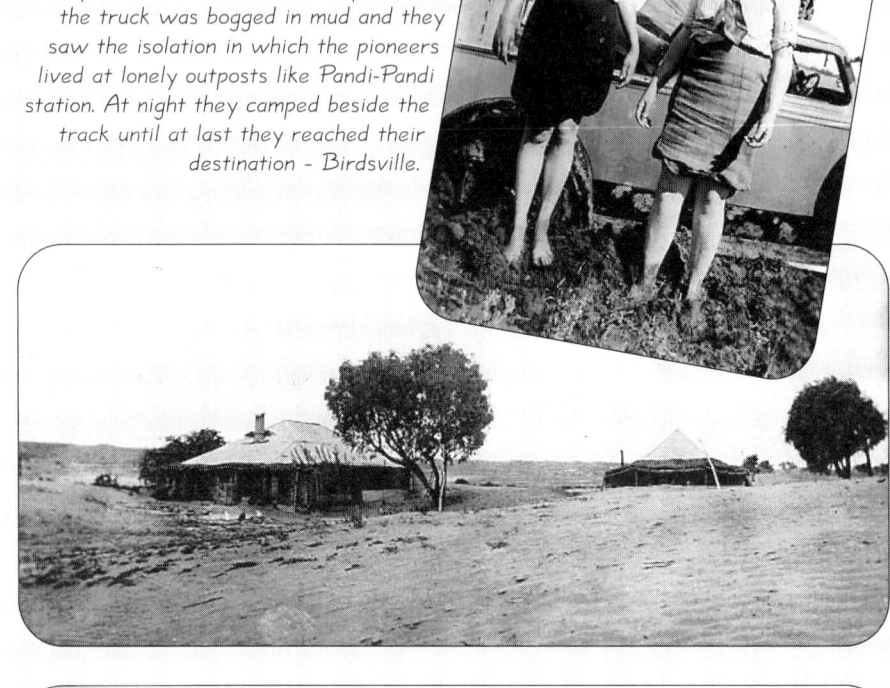

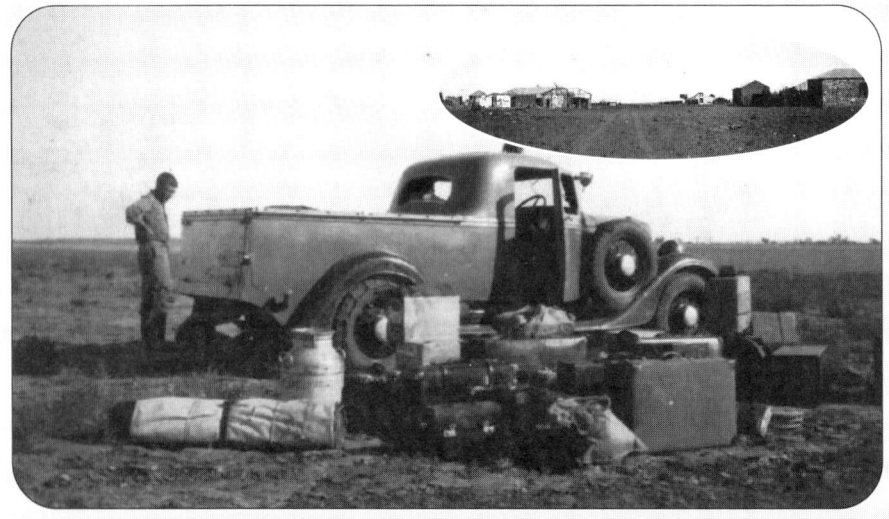

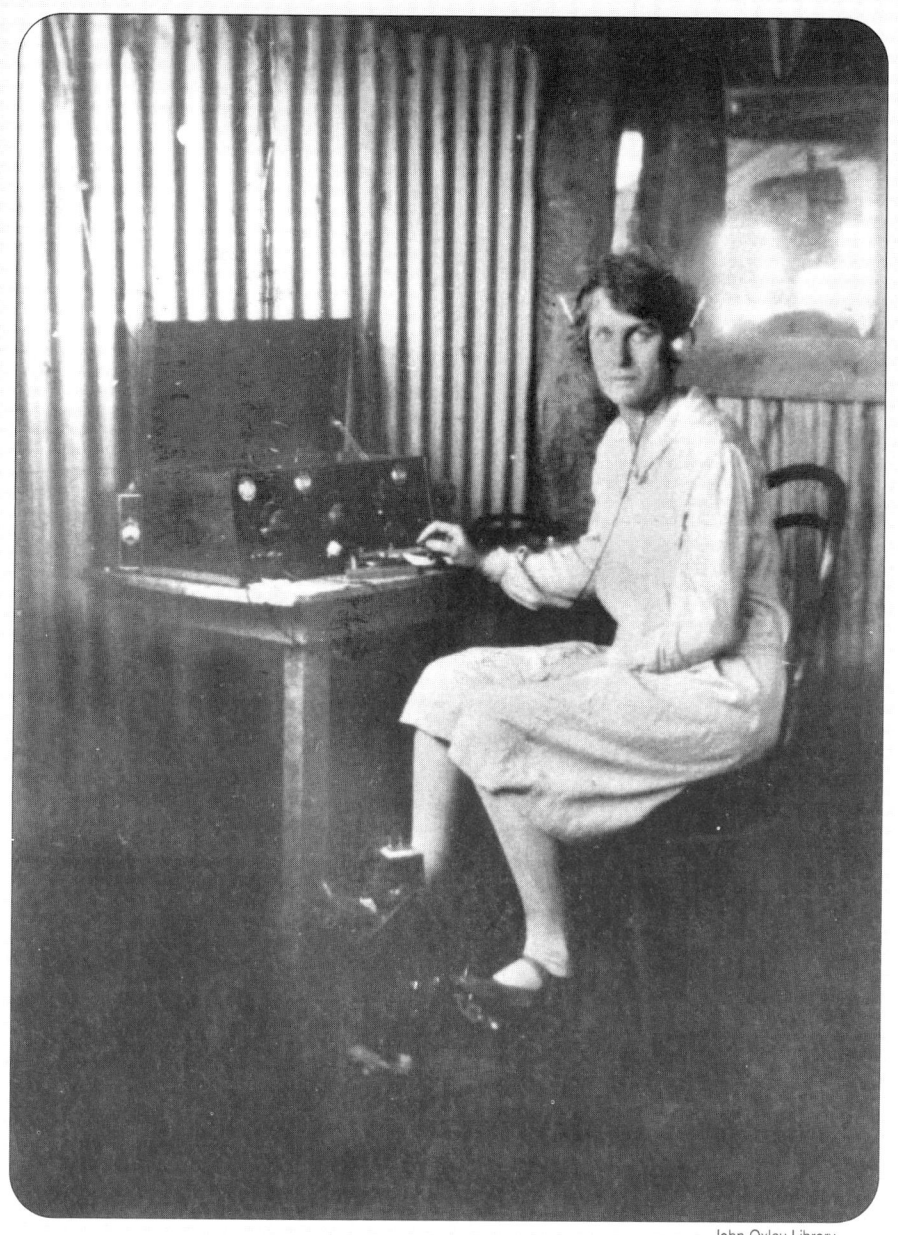

John Oxley Library

Mrs Gertrude Rothery of Augustus Downs in 1929 sent the first ever successful transmission from her homestead to Cloncurry.
"Greetings by wireless service from Augustus Downs. First station installed. Manager, family and station deeply appreciate service rendered."
The message was sent on to Flynn in Sydney.

Right: Jean White, the world's first female flying doctor, photographed in 1938.

Centre: Jean's plane after it crashed on Cocomungin Island, far north Queensland, in January 1939.

Below: Jean White enjoyed the friendship and fellowship of the AIM family. At this picnic we see (from left) Jean, Mrs Simpson, Fred McKay, Flying Doctor Gordon Alberry, John Flynn and his wife Jean.

John Oxley Library

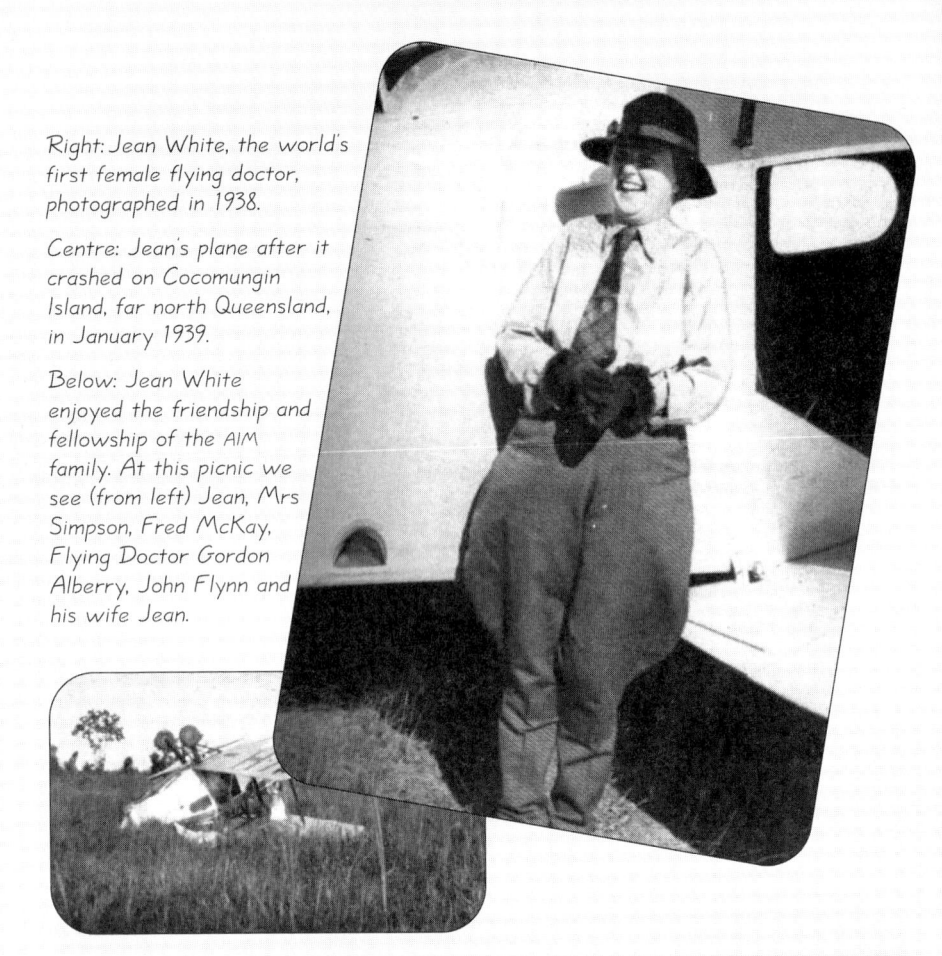

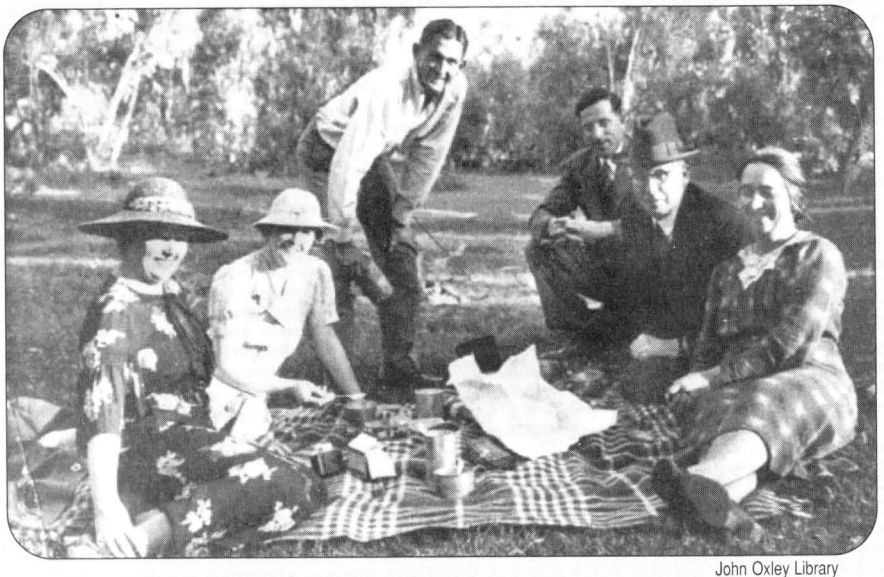

Flynn had written to Sir Josiah earlier:

> For eleven years I have been organising this movement, and have steadily refused to become a mere beggar. I have contended that, if we "lifted up" the ideal, men of wide vision and statesmanlike thinking would rally to our side and constrain their fellows to do big things.

The publication of Sir Josiah's letter had that exact effect, and donations began to pour in to "Sister Kinnear's Appeal" for furnishings and equipment. Sir Josiah was a respected lawyer, the leader of the Adelaide Bar, and had served a term as Attorney-General. Being so prominent, others followed his example and gave support to the concept of a hospital at Innamincka.

Minnie Kinnear went for a second term of service to The Mitchell Home, Beltana. "It seems like a suburban posting after Innamincka," she commented. She maintained her interest in the progress of the hospital at Innamincka. Her many friends in the Channel Country kept her posted and she shared some of their letters and concerns with the AIM. For example, in March 1925 and a year after Josiah Symon's gift, she sent this extract from a letter sent to her about a man who had to be evacuated from Tragedy Corner:

> They had to take one of the men down to Port Augusta hospital [530 miles]. The doctor there says he has a very bad form of fever and has very little hope for him. The man seemed to be just about done when he passed here, the first 100 of the 530 miles. He did not know much and had had it [the fever] nine days when they started out. He is a stranger in a strange land; he landed from Ireland a short time ago and came straight up here to Innamincka... The hospital would get plenty of use if it was going now.

Minnie sent comments with this letter in an effort to ginger up the plans for the hospital:

> Since my return a year ago, I have frequently received letters from people within one or two hundred miles of the proposed Nursing Home there, and they are hoping to see "the walls of the hospital springing up soon".

> The 530 miles that man would have had to travel are in very rough country, as I know. Part of the journey to the railway would be over sand-hills and part would have to be covered in a camel buggy. Over sandy country coconut matting is laid in places to enable the motors to get through and one can only travel at 10 miles per hour. Then when the railway is reached, one may have to wait a couple of days for a train and travel 220 miles further on to Port Augusta.
>
> A nursing home would save much suffering and some lives as well. We have dreamed dreams and seen visions of it for some months now, and £2000 for building purposes and £450 for furnishings are available. It would be good news to know that a small building with plenty of veranda space would be ready soon to accommodate these needy, uncomplaining pioneers.

Flynn shared her impatience. In his reply, he fumed: "My Board is anxious to have the Innamincka Hospital completed at the earliest possible moment, but then enumerates two pages of reasons why it has to be delayed."

Flynn's vision was always in advance of his Board. However, he went ahead and sketched out plans based on Minnie's advice for "wide verandah space" and other suggestions. The result was a hospital very like that he had built himself with bleeding hands in Alice Springs, a hospital with sleeping quarters upstairs and the business end downstairs, and an underground cellar for storing supplies.

Even when building started, progress was slow because materials had to be carted by camel and truck over the tortuous track from Broken Hill to Innamincka. Two further Border Sisters had to go out, the first being Sister Grant and then Sister Clare Stewart.

The sparkling new Elizabeth Symon Nursing Home was opened in May 1929. The local policeman, Jack Ridge, has left us a description:

> On the day of the opening, I put on full uniform to try to make the occasion more formal. None of the kids in that locality seemed to have ever seen a policeman in uniform

before, because wherever I went they all followed, even looking through windows and calling to their mates, "He's coming out" this or that door. The uniform was a much better drawcard than any other part of the festivities. The Nursing Home was declared open by the Reverend Andrew Barber, of Melbourne, who was staying with me at the time. Sisters Clare Stewart and Elsbeth Edgar were the first to staff it. There was much typhoid fever about at that time, and the two Sisters and I did six months straight nursing. I buried a number of people in that area. They were buried either in their swag or I made a sort of coffin from the grog cases— the only sawn timber available.

Minnie's dream of a hospital had at last come true, and on an even grander scale than she had envisioned. In fact, an enthusiastic reporter labelled it "the best building in the Inland" and many locals agreed. Besides smart bedrooms for the Sisters upstairs, a "Blue Room" and a "Mauve Room", it had water laid on from its own well and windmill, a real bathroom, and the wide, shaded verandahs that Minnie had insisted upon. Thick concrete walls helped to keep out the heat. To facilitate effective nursing there was a general ward, a dispensary and even the dental chair that Minnie had requested.

With the hospital up and running, the Mantle of Safety in its wider sense soon invaded the region. Within a year the nurses were learning Morse code and using Traeger's transceivers to contact the Flying Doctor at Cloncurry for advice. No longer need they diagnose and treat everything by themselves unaided and in dreadful isolation.

And that same year, 1934, Doctor Jock Rossell made the first emergency Flying Doctor trip to Innamincka and thereby fulfilled another of Minnie's dreams.

Even though Jean Finlayson and Minnie Kinnear had nursed in gruelling conditions without hospitals, their experiences and advice contributed directly to fine hospitals being built subsequently.

* * * *

AND HOW DID the Innamincka Hospital fare?

At first it was a very visible success. Sir Josiah Symon was pleased with the sterling work done there, and it proved to be an oasis of mercy. Proudly, he gave out Flynn's reports of its progress to family and friends until his death in 1934.

Flynn's nurses did an exceptional job over the years and were respected, indeed loved, by that rough community. They treated sores and wounds, delivered babies, extracted teeth, fought various diseases and undertook for all the medical challenges, but in addition gave Sunday School lessons, battled heat and flies and dust storms, hosted dances and helped to organise Christmas celebrations and the Picnic Races.

A run of terrible droughts then devastated the Innamincka region and huge dust storms blew across the deserts. After one, the Sisters described how they would shelter from it, by sitting with their heads as well as their food under the tablecloth. And when the storm has passed, the dust on the hospital floors was so thick it was "all in ripples like a beach, just as though the tide had washed it". These droughts hammered the region economically.

The Innamincka Hospital served the region admirably as its only medical facility until 1951 when it closed down, because of a thinning population and the availability of the RFDS. It had been far more than just a hospital, as Fred McKay commented: "The home was not just a medical centre but an important social centre as well. It was a place to read newspapers or to have tea and a chat in a comfortable chair. The Sisters stood for good bush hospitality."

While some of the cattle stations have closed down as a result of the droughts, Innamincka is still one of the S. Kidman & Co. properties and considered to be one of the best arid-lands cattle properties in Australia.

In recent years a dramatic increase in tourism has seen the fortunes of the region undergo a revival—a modern hotel and store were built in 1972 and are doing well. And the Elizabeth Symon Nursing Home has been restored with the help of a massive fundraising effort spearheaded by *Australian Geographic* magazine. It now serves as the National Parks Visitor Centre and has displays in the old general ward that illustrate the development of the Nursing Home. It even boasts some of the uniforms and equipment used by Flynn's nurses. Perhaps closer to Flynn's heart, it has a first aid centre to service the 30,000 annual visitors and the local inhabitants. Furthermore, the Patrol Padres sleep there when in the region, thereby retaining some links with Flynn's dreams.

Perhaps the trend to rediscover Australian history will result in greater appreciation also for Minnie Kinnear, that tiny slim woman who served the outback so courageously but with scant official recognition.

Both Minnie and Jean had to make epic journeys at times simply to reach patients, or to take them to a doctor, using whatever means of transport they could. This has always been a feature of Flynn's nurses, that they were prepared to rough it to arrive at their destination. In the following chapter we will take a brief look at some other outback journeys undertaken by Flynn's nurses.

5

Snippets of Journeys

John Flynn had a saying: "Half the challenge of serving people in the outback involves getting there, and the other half involves staying there."

Transport from the hospital to patients was a challenge for the early nurses and the ability to ride a horse was a prerequisite. He often told the story of Sister Bett on an emergency call at night peering for indistinct camel pads by walking with a lantern for hours in front of a coach and horses. As the inland developed, so too did the transport options available to Flynn's nurses.

* * * *

Motorcars began as very unreliable and difficult to use in a land where smooth roads did not exist. May Gillespie (Maranboy, 1917–18) records what they were like to travel in:

> Judge Bevan's motorcar was mounted on a truck in front of the train and we occupied it. At Katherine the car was taken off the truck and we motored on to Maranboy. The track was very bumpy and sandy and progress was slow. At each stretch of sand the car was stopped. One end of a long rope was tied to a tree and the other was attached to a winch on the front of the car, which progressed as the rope was wound onto the drum… The winch was severely tested when the wheels sank deep into the sand and there was only one suitable tree nearby. We waited with bated breath as the rope took the strain and the engine made a high-pitched whine. Suddenly there was a loud crack. But the motor had not come free, instead the tree had been uprooted! We resorted to the tedious work of digging the wheels free and manhandling the motor forwards.

Many of Flynn's nurses were city girls and the romance of trekking through the bush excited them. Elizabeth Burchill and Ina Currey served at Innamincka from 1930 to 1932. Ina wrote to Flynn to describe their trip out using both cars and camels:

> It certainly is a justly famous drive; the Aboriginal boy sat on the running board to tell the mailman the track. We wound between the sand hills and every now and again we'd CHARGE a sand drift, change the gears, and swoop down on the other side. I never imagined a car could perform such acrobatics. The radiator boiled and bubbled till we thought we'd go up in smoke, but it was all tremendous fun.
>
> We made our camp inside "The Cobbler" [a parched desert area] and we almost felt as though we'd stepped straight out of the Arabian Nights with our camels humped on the far side of the fire and our Aboriginal boys moving about them. We unrolled our swags and went to sleep under the wide and starry sky.

In 1936, Fred McKay took two young nurses, Alice "Andy" Anderson and Lillian Cooper, to Birdsville in his truck. Fresh from the city, they took pleasure in the novelty of their experiences. Alice recalls:

> Lillian and I enjoyed our nights in the open. The air is usually very dry and a tent is not necessary, so we slept in swags beside the track. A canvas sheet is spread on the ground, then the bed made up with pillows and blankets. The ground sheet is folded up from the feet and down from the head to form a sort of envelope.
>
> As we lay there, in our swags, the nights were lovely. The sky was like black velvet and the stars seemed somehow bigger and brighter. We learned the meaning of starlight because the nights never seemed to get really dark.
>
> The roads, mainly faint bush tracks, were very rough and travelling slow. We got bogged in a creek one evening and spent the next day trying to dig and winch the truck out, but only moved six feet. Fortunately, there was a station homestead about a mile or so away and when they saw lights for the second night they realised someone was in trouble and came to help. With their block and tackle, they got us out in only half an hour. They made pungent remarks

about city drivers who ran into a bog when there was a well-marked track around it – in fact two *very* faint wheel tracks on some very hard earth. Poor Fred was most embarrassed.

From Betoota, the regular track to Birdsville was cut by flooding, so Fred enlisted the services of Joe Hagan, the packhorse mailman, to guide us. Suddenly the trip became incredibly rough. Joe knew more about guiding horses than motors because motors cannot simply step over gibbers. Fred had to be constantly on the alert because there was the danger of a cracked sump going over large rocks. We seemed to twist and turn an awful lot, but Fred had to follow Joe's leading regardless. Only later did we discover why we had woven such a weird and wonderful track, when Joe could not see a horse grazing just a stone's throw away. He was incredibly short sighted! Instead of fixing his sight on distant objects and setting a straight course, he had steered haphazardly around nearby features—and where he led, we had to follow.

Eventually we had to abandon the truck and complete our journey to Birdsville by boat, the Diamantina having burst its banks.

When we arrived at the opposite side, there was no motor to take us into Birdsville itself, so Fred fired off the shotgun hoping that someone in the town would come and pick us up. Thankfully, it worked. The truck was only brought across the Diamantina days later.

Lillian and Alice had other misadventures with transport during their service at Birdsville, including being stuck in the mud. "On the way the utility bogged. The lass decided to have her baby there and then—so she was delivered in the back of the utility, in a bog, by moonlight."

Lillian had not finished with boats in the desert either. She married Peter Stevenson, then bookkeeper at Glengyle station, at the end of her term of service. When their first child was due in 1940, the region was flooded once again and it was impossible to use the roads in or out. In desperation, Peter rowed her up the swollen Georgina River and Bob Gaffney took over from Cuttaburra and boated her to the Birdsville Track. Ken Crombie, in the mail truck, battled through the mud and sludge to Marree. Others helped until her colleague from Birdsville, Sister 'Andy' Anderson, met her and drove to Broken Hill. A long train ride eventually brought her to Brisbane where the lusty baby William was delivered successfully. Few babies have had a more varied journey before seeing the light of day!

Trains were more reliable than cars in the early years, but scarcely more comfortable. Sister Dunlop (Maranboy 1920–22) wrote: "Leaping Lena, as the train was called, jerked when starting off sidings and nearly threw us off our seats, which caused the name I guess."

Indeed, there was no really comfortable form of transport in the bush such as we have nowadays. Bruce Plowman, Flynn's first Patrol Padre, commented on the hardness of the seats of bush vehicles in *Camel Pads:* "It was commonly reported that passengers developed corns on a part of their anatomy where no corns ought to grow."

Occasionally nurses travelled on camels, but these would sway to and fro and could cause queasiness. Furthermore, they were cantankerous, described by Jean Finlayson as "unpleasant beasts and dangerous at both ends".

Flynn always tried to improve things and kept an eye on modern developments, including the use of his beloved aeroplanes. However, these were small craft and easily buffeted by winds and storms. Sister Joyce Falconbridge (Wimmera Home, 1937–39), who had been advised to go to a warmer climate for the sake of her health, recalls:

> I told the doctor where I was going and he said "Good heavens, woman, I told you to go to a hot climate, I didn't tell you to go to hell"...We flew to Daly Waters in a four-seater. I was terrified and the flight was bumpy. The navigator was reading a book titled when the *World Turned Upside Down*. I was crying when we arrived.

Marathon journeys were necessary at times, not only for nurses, but also for women on properties. Elsie Bohning and her mother Esther took charge of the first trainload of stock from Alice Springs to Adelaide, despite opposition from officials who doubted they could manage. Just twenty years old and attractive, Elsie was popular with the press when the two women eventually made it to Adelaide. While she enjoyed the sights of a big city, Elsie was soon ready to return to the bush. Not only did mother and daughter succeed in this venture, but other similar feats followed and they won renown as the "Petticoat Drovers". Elsie was a great supporter of Flynn's work and proclaimed its value in articles and letters. She wrote for the *Northern Territory Times*, calling herself the "Little Bush Maid".

The mail and also the supplies upon which the bush depended could have very mixed journeys. Ron Easy describes the situation on Rockhampton Downs in the late twenties and early thirties:

> All supplies came once a year, about April, by horse team. They arrived by ship in Burketown, on the Gulf, and were picked up from there. The wagons took about six weeks to get through. Strange things happened to foodstuffs!
>
> There was a six-weekly mail service from Camooweal to Boorooloola that called at Alroy en route. My parents' transport was a buggy pulled by two draught horses, so the round trip to get their mail took about a week. Mum liked going for the mail as it gave her the opportunity to sleep in a real bed, in a house. Most of all, she was able to enjoy the company of ladies at Alroy.

Similarly, supplies for nursing homes could have a tortuous passage. Sister Betty Wood (Wimmera Home, 1926–28) described the journey that their stores took:

> We got our stores in twice a year. They had to be taken 80 miles down the river by boat and then 80 miles by donkey wagon. And you can imagine what the stores were like when they did arrive, as they were a week on the boat and a fortnight on the wagon in the boiling sun. The boat service was terribly uncertain and I remember the Christmas ham arriving in April one year.

But of all the journeys taken by Flynn's nurses and their goods and chattels, perhaps none could match that of Grace Francis and Catherine Boyd. Their epic begins in the next chapter.

6

Birdsville Needs a Hospital— Grace Francis

Birdsville is one of the most isolated outposts on earth. It lies on the edge of the Simpson Desert to the west and Sturt's Stony Desert to the east and is battered by dust storms and baking heat. Its famous mailman, Tom Kruse, recalls being told when he first went there he was lucky because the temperature had fallen below 120 degrees for the first time for days. Prolonged periods with temperatures above that have been reported.

Why Birdsville should become established at all in such hostile environs is a bit of an enigma. Captain Charles Sturt, the famous explorer, made no bones about the unpleasant nature of the region during his search for an inland sea in 1845. Then followed the disastrous Burke and Wills expedition in 1860. However, some adventurous souls wondered if cattle might not be established on big runs in the semi-desert lands and ventured in along the river channels—the Diamantina and Cooper being significant in this. Both are capricious and water flowed only sporadically, but it transpired there was unusually good rainfall and promising feed for animal stock for a few years in the 1860s, and again in the 1870s, allowing some cattle stations to become established. These unusual years were interspersed by the more usual dry conditions and droughts that decimated the livestock. Nevertheless, some rugged individualists hung on, hoping for conditions to improve, while others adjusted to the harsh environment and wrenched a tenuous livelihood from it. But these hardy pioneers needed a distribution centre for their supplies, and there was also a need for the Government of Queensland to tax and police the region. The centre chosen for these activities was at Birdsville, on a stock route near to a ford over the Diamantina and 12 kilometres from the border with South Australia. The main streets of Birdsville dissolved into sand dunes and gibbers once outside the town.

In pioneering days, medical help was available at Birdsville only if a visiting doctor happened to be passing through. One such rare occasion was in 1892 when Mrs Bell was expecting her first child. A cooperative policeman took the precaution of locking up the doctor on some trivial charge to ensure both his presence and his sobriety at the birth. The policeman's motives were not entirely without self-interest; too many times when things went wrong medically the community looked to him to help and he would do his best, using common sense and an old medical book he owned. Sometimes the patient recovered and sometimes he died, in which case filling in forms regarding the cause of death was problematical for the policeman. But in the case of Mrs Bell, with a proper doctor attending, a healthy baby was born.

Not everyone was as fortunate as Mrs Bell and there were many tragedies over the years. Accounts of these and other problems associated with inadequate medical help in Birdsville kept coming to Flynn.

So the compassionate Flynn began to put money aside with which to build a cottage hospital in Birdsville when the call came, as he felt sure it would because the need was great, and it would be too difficult for the Government to build and staff an official hospital. The locals, though, were inclined to put their faith in the Government building a "proper hospital with a doctor attending" rather than the nursing home that Flynn could offer.

In 1921, after an unaided confinement, Mary Smith was delivered of beautiful twins—Dorothy Ellen and William Patrick. Her husband Samuel, along with a neighbour and a visiting relative, assisted at the birth. This was a significant moment in Birdsville's history as Samuel had been the first white child born there and the twins symbolised continuity and permanence. But the tragedy that followed was in a strange way to prove even more significant—the twins died within a month. Perhaps they died of the Spanish influenza carried by a friend who visited.

No sooner had the tiny bodies of the twins been laid in the windswept cemetery than the grieving community stopped wavering and approached Flynn to establish a cottage hospital there as soon as possible, believing that his nurses could have saved the little mites. Besides, they pondered, what of the next man or woman to fall sick in the region? At least some lives could be saved and much suffering alleviated if Flynn built a cottage hospital: who could predict how many more years would pass before the Government acted?

Meanwhile tragedies kept occurring. Constable John Gurn lodged this report of events at Annadale station on 23rd January 1922:

> Left at daylight and arrived at Annadale station at 6 p.m. having ridden 50 miles that day. Dug grave by lantern light. Next morning shown dead bodies of two male children on single bed. Temperature approximately 120 degrees Fahrenheit. Buried bodies. Took statement. Rode back to Birdsville then rode model-T Ford to Boulia 250 miles to send telegram to Cloncurry police.

The grave Constable Gurn dug is still there. Once again, the Birdsville community believed that Willie (aged 8) and Darwin (aged 2) need not have died if proper nursing care had been available. The calls to Flynn for help became strident.

Flynn wanted to comply right away, but realised the awesome challenges that had to be faced by the first nurses. He would need experienced women tough enough to survive primitive conditions and extremes of nature; women resourceful enough to make do without doctor, wireless, telephone or aeroplane available, yet compassionate enough to serve the locals and win their hearts. So this would be a particularly tough assignment and he did not advertise the position in the media. He wanted to hand pick the first nurses if possible, because the success or failure of their mission would determine the future of his hospital there. But whom could he approach? Enter Grace Francis, a committed Christian nurse with whom he had been corresponding about the work of the AIM. She had the qualities he sought. He decided to ask her.

* * * *

Ida Grace Francis was born at Bega in New South Wales on 22nd July 1892.

She began her nursing training in Gympie General Hospital, Queensland, in 1909, where she proved that she was well suited to the nursing profession and from which she issued with outstanding qualifications. Furthermore, she saw nursing not simply as a job but as a vocation, and believed it to be her calling from God.

Volunteering for service with the Army, she served for two gruelling and often traumatic years in World War I, both in England and in France. She demonstrated courage, commitment, compassion and character. The very rugged and difficult conditions of the war provided her with that special preparation Flynn was looking for. Furthermore, she ardently supported his visions about the long-term need for a wireless network and "air doctors". A woman of outstanding intelligence and organising skills, she would be capable of helping to establish wireless at Birdsville—if only he could launch something. He had already resolved that radio communications must become available in Birdsville if its isolation was to be broken.

Flynn approached Sister Francis with the proposal that she and a nursing colleague pioneer a hospital at Birdsville. The need was too urgent for Flynn to try and build one, which could take years as all materials had to be carted in hundreds of kilometres by camels along the Birdsville Track, so he proposed starting in the old Royal Hotel, crudely built of hewn stone and mud and now derelict.

Grace Francis did not accept at once, realising the need for a colleague of similar determined outlook and nursing skills. She approached her young friend Sister Catherine Boyd, who gallantly accepted the stern challenge.

The two nurses left Brisbane on 7th September 1923. Birdsville was 1800 kilometres away and the final legs were to be along rough desert tracks.

Sister Francis has left us a diary. In it she made bland, underscored statements about this gruelling journey, including:

> SEPTEMBER 1923.
>
> 7th: Left Brisbane at 2 p.m. Mr Walker and Mr Galloway had some difficulty getting stretchers on board for us in case of camping out on the Birdsville side of the journey.

> 10th: Left [Charleville] by the mail lorry at about 9 a.m. We had the best seats available in front and changed every 10 or 20 miles as one seat was very low and we got cramped up a bit. We found it very hot as the day wore on and, not having a hood in the lorry, we tried to keep our umbrellas up – they turned inside out a few times. The men sat on top of a mountain of mailbags. We stopped frequently to put letters into a lonely little letterbox by the way, usually made of a kerosene tin.
>
> We lunched at "Jack-on-the-Rocks", so called on account of a man named Jack who died there. Quite a young woman, three children and a governess live there. It seems so desolate, dry and hot, that I don't know how they exist, but they seem quite happy.
>
> After leaving, we crossed the Bulgaroo Plains, two miles of black soil recently traversed by a mob of cattle in the wet, so we had a very rough ride.
>
> We dropped a passenger in the middle of the plain, his sole luggage being a bundle tied up in a large handkerchief, and a catalogue. His camp, he told us, was nine miles off where he had a wife and children. I felt very sorry for him but he seemed quite at home and happy.
>
> 11th: Arrived at Windorah at 3 p.m. and came to McPhillamy's Hotel. We expect to see a car to meet us from Birdsville any day. Failing that we will take the coach on the 20th.

However, the car from Birdsville did not arrive. An adjustment made in the hotel was to banish, temporarily, the talking cockatoo; his language was considered unfit for the Sisters' ears.

Rather than sit idly by, the Sisters visited each person in the vicinity and soon their medical skills were called upon. Grace put in two temporary fillings. Then a more worrying case presented itself:

> 14th: The Police Sergeant asked us to go and see his sick child today. The little chap (4 years) looks very ill.
>
> 15th: Sergeant's child looking very bad indeed. Have advised them to take him to Jundah Hospital (60 miles).

> Temperature of 102 degrees. *Looks like typhoid fever.* Attended 15 others—a dental case; one extraction.
>
> Visited Sergeant's child again at 8 p.m. He is still looking, and is, very ill. One of us may travel to Jundah with him.
>
> 16th: Left for Jundah with Freddie Stokes at 8 a.m. arrived there 2 p.m. Interviewed the doctor and then took the patient to the hospital. The parents were very upset when doctor pronounced typhoid fever.

But the child survived. Her early diagnosis and advice to take the child to hospital without doubt saved his life. This gift of diagnosis was to save more lives in Birdsville.

> 18th: A car drove up which turned out to be Mr Brook and Mr Reese from Birdsville, come to meet us. I nearly hugged them! We are glad to see the car for we did not like the thought of the coach.

These two men were both experienced bushmen, especially Lou Reese, who had a good reputation in the Inland. Lou had guided and befriended John Flynn a dozen years previously when Flynn travelled the Birdsville Track. He would now carefully watch the Sisters in that casual yet penetrating way that typifies the true bushman. If he liked what he saw, they could count on his personal support and influence, which would greatly facilitate their acceptance in Birdsville.

Almost immediately Lou Reese had the opportunity to observe Sister Grace in action. That very night there was an emergency call.

> 19th: Were called out to a patient 20 miles away at midnight. The road was easy to follow to Old Galway station but after that we had to follow a sheep pad. We reached the camp at about 2 a.m., found Mrs Dare in no immediate danger but thought it better to get her away to a doctor. Got back to Windorah at 5 a.m. and after fixing up the patient went to bed for a while.
>
> At 4 p.m. Mrs Dare did not seem at all well and as we were to leave for Birdsville tomorrow, think we will take her to Jundah.

> 20th: Took Mrs Dare to Jundah last night and took her to Nurse Grant. The doctor lives just opposite so she will be all right.

Lou Reese was suitably impressed. The cheerful attitude of the two Sisters despite discomforts on the road also augured well for their pioneering in Birdsville. In fact, he liked them so much he decided to take them to meet his wife and family on the way in.

> 22nd: Left Beetoota at 8 a.m. The roads were exceedingly bad. Such sand-hills and gibbers, the roughest road I have ever travelled. The country seemed to get more bare and timberless.
> We landed at the Reese's at about 8 p.m. and gave them a big surprise, being the first visitors (women) they had ever had!
>
> 23rd: Early in the a.m. I heard the chatter of the gins [Aboriginal women] and Mrs Reese brought in four of them to see "two feller white woman". They filed in one at a time and peered down into my face and seemed to be enjoying the joke very much.
> After 11 a.m. tea we made a start for the last 38 miles for Birdsville, crossing the border fence at 3 p.m. and arriving in Birdsville at 4 p.m.

It had taken sixteen days to cover the 1800 kilometres from Brisbane to Birdsville.

The Sisters had a minimum of luggage with them when they arrived. Their main supplies, including furniture, drugs, etc., had been sent via South Australia and camel train as there was no luggage route between Brisbane and Birdsville. Nobody had any clear idea of when they could expect it to arrive. They were disappointed that it had not preceded them, but Flynn had made arrangements that they were to stay at the Birdsville Hotel until it came.

With Lou Reese to guide them, they went down to look over the old Royal Hotel that Flynn had hired to serve as the first AIM hospital in Birdsville. In keeping with his philosophy of it serving the community socially and spiritually as well as medically, it was to be named the "Brisbane Home" and not a hospital at all—

although the locals ignored Flynn's name for the most part. It was an old mud and hewn-stone building with wide clay verandas, whose tin roof was held up with crooked poles. The mud walling would be unsound if rained on directly, but the overhanging verandah would act like an umbrella to protect it. Besides, it seldom rained in Birdsville.

Expecting to find it filthy inside, they were delighted to find the people of Birdsville had swept it out and had whitewashed the walls—so it had a pleasantly fresh appearance. It comprised two large rooms and four smaller ones and a veranda floor made from bottle tops.

As they walked around, Catherine looked upwards and exclaimed, "We'll not be robbed of seeing the stars at night." She pointed to a series of gaping holes in the roof.

"It'll do the job just fine. It's good-oh," Grace pronounced, to Lou's amusement and pleasure. If the Sisters had proven fussy they would have lost local support very quickly. As it was, he had already fielded negative comments from some of the locals: "Bloody missionaries. We don't want any bloody missionaries around here." He gently communicated to the Sisters that there were those who held that view.

Grace was a bit perplexed to learn from him that there were some strong critics of their cottage hospital. Well then, they would simply have to win the critics over! In a small community, criticism could easily result in rejection of their services, making their efforts futile.

They returned to the hotel. The manager, Mrs Gaffney, was suffering with rotten teeth and wanted to become their first patient. It was too late to do anything further that night though. The two women were exhausted, so had supper and went to bed:

> 24th: A heavy wind and dust blew up during the night. The house rattled like a matchbox. We could not sleep very much. The people are giving a little welcome to us tonight. We had a little walk to the water hole with Mr Reese in the afternoon.

Their inspection of the water supply had been because the Sisters needed to know where to fetch their water. Grace was disquieted that the water was murky "until the Diamantina floods, then it gets flushed out and freshened up". She noted, but said nothing at the time, the animal remains that lay in the channel along which the fresh water would come rushing. At a more opportune time something would have to be done about that for the sake of public health!

They attended the friendly gathering that evening. "Quite a large gathering to welcome us. I was surprised to see so many women; there being nine in all, and this is not all of the residents. Dancing was kept up until 12.30 p.m. I managed to say a few words of appreciation."

Lou Reese, meanwhile, told everyone what "good sorts" the two Sisters were and how effectively they had cared for the sick during the journey out. He wrote in the same vein to Flynn, declaring, "If ever angels came on earth, I would say these are two." Flynn was delighted with this ringing endorsement from a tough old bushman and quoted it extensively in his talks and sermons as well as in his magazine, the *Inlander*.

Mrs Gaffney had a problem with the Sisters staying at the hotel for a prolonged time, though; the annual races, due to be held the following month, had become a big event, and the hotel had been booked out. Where could the two nurses stay during race week? Boldly, they decided to stay at the old Royal Hotel despite having no furniture yet. They had their two camp stretchers after all and would still eat at the hotel until they could organise cooking facilities for themselves. Mrs Gaffney was relieved by the decision and offered them two spare mattresses from the hotel to tide them over until their own arrived and a broom and shovel to sweep out the inches of dust that blew in during dust storms. Thus it was that the two nurses planned their occupation of Brisbane Home. Which room would they sleep in? They chose the old bar. They scrounged some boxes to use as chairs and constructed a "table" from rickety crates.

Sister Grace next set about winning the confidence of Birdsville. She started visiting extensively, finding the locals to be friendly and enjoying a yarn. She tended any sick in their own homes as there was nowhere suitable at the hotel and they had not yet set up their hospital. Besides, people felt less threatened to begin with, less intimidated, in their own homes rather than in a hospital.

The two Sisters were keen to launch something spiritual as soon as possible. On their first Sunday after their arrival in Birdsville, the 30th September, they bemoaned: "We missed having a piano, and besides could not use the hotel." Patience was needed. They had noticed an old piano in a shed by the Royal Hotel, but this belonged to the previous owner. Grace wrote at once to Flynn asking whether it could be purchased for the AIM. She pointed out that entertainments were few in the bush and a piano would draw people to their home, not just for church services but also for social singing. As soon as Flynn received the communication he concurred and acted, but that still took a while.

Ken Griffin, the schoolteacher, invited them to visit his school the following day, Monday 1st October. This visit was to prove significant in their work for the region. They found twenty-eight lively pupils and they offered to give sewing lessons once a week to the girls, who were very excited at the prospect. The lessons were to prove very popular.

However, it was as the children tried to read that Grace was shocked. Most of them had visual impairment to a greater or lesser degree. Her cursory observations suggested sandy blight was the primary cause.

She discussed this with Ken Griffin. He admitted children often arrived at school with discharging eyes and usually he would try and help them by giving them an eyebath with salt water or weak bicarbonate of soda solution. This had not been very successful but it had been the best he had been able to do.

"You have done well," Grace reassured him, "but in fact they need treatment with the proper eye salve. Unfortunately it has not yet arrived, but as soon as it does we'll help lift your burden and treat them with it ourselves. Some of them have sores and teeth that need attention also, but the sandy blight is the greatest immediate danger they face."

Her diary tersely records their settling in and how their services began to be called upon:

October 1923.

> 1st: Filled two teeth for Dorothy Gaffney. She also has a boil on her face which I dressed.
>
> 2nd: Moved down to the hospital to sleep.
>
> 3rd: Treated David Hagan with small pustules on hands. We are working under difficulties without drug supplies. Two other children with toothache had a temporary filling put in. Played bridge and ping pong with Mr and Mrs Brook and Mr Griffin. Also had tea with them.
>
> 5th: Mr Reese sent an Aboriginal boy in with a horse to be raffled for the hospital! Marree coach left today. Mr Russell, the driver, had a septic finger which I dressed two or three times; it looked much better when he left.
>
> 9th: A heavy dust storm again today. Trees are flying everywhere. Managed to get a bit of practice on the old piano. Mrs Brook loaned us a kettle and teapot to make ourselves a cup of afternoon tea. She also gives me a cup of [goat's] milk every day. Everybody is talking races. The women are getting ready for a fancy dress ball. Dorothy Gaffney still having ingrown toenails treated. The storm went down about 6 p.m. and a nice cool night followed.

The Sisters also let it be known that they would join in with community games and other activities. To be fully accepted, and to be able to play their social and spiritual roles most effectively, they needed to be seen as "one of us". They swam with locals, went horse riding and played ping-pong, etc. They also joined in their picnics. At one of these Grace won second prize in the wheelbarrow race, which indicates her great sense of fun. In all her work and interrelating with the community she displayed good humour, friendliness, kindness, thoughtfulness and sympathy. Within a short time the Sisters were liked and accepted.

All the while, they were stultified in their socialising at the Royal by a lack of proper furniture. For example, during the races, a number of folk dropped in to meet them and to have a chat. "We had only boxes to sit on and all manner of vessels to drink from."

By the 21st October, Grace decided their primitive conditions might not be suitable for adults but could still host Sunday School for children. Feeling that they were becoming trusted sufficiently, she mooted the concept in the community. It met with general support.

The lack of proper furniture meant also that their treatment room was inadequate, especially for dentistry:

> 27th: A very hot day. Mrs McAuley came in with toothache, could not manage to extract as she pulled away. Only having her sitting on a box without support for the head, it was a difficult job. I hate to let her go with the tooth not out. She has suffered great pain. She is to come back in a day or two. Mr Lee and Mr Griffin called about 5 p.m. and we had a game of ping-pong. After tea we drove a little way along the road with them and walked back.
>
> 8th: Sunday. We held our first Sunday School class. Today seven children attended. This morning a patient, Mr West [drover] came in with an abscess on his face and as I had only scissors, had to open it with them. It was superficial and was very easy, the pus just poured out and gave him such relief that when we arranged two boxes and got him lying down and a good hot foment on the face, he went to sleep for an hour or so.

In terms of medical help, the Sisters rapidly became "it". For example, in Birdsville there was no visiting doctor to wait for and the nearest telephone to ring up for advice or help was a tortuous 400 kilometres away. The Sisters were forced to make decisions that took their breath away. Grace's gifting in diagnosis and her wide experience during the war and afterwards proved invaluable.

Chatting with their sewing and Sunday School classes, the Sisters discovered the children had never experienced a Christmas tree with presents and a Father Christmas. Despite living in such primitive conditions themselves, they determined to organise Christmas festivities for the local children. They set to writing letters – asking their home churches to send parcels for under the Christmas tree. They baked and sewed themselves and enlisted the help of other women to do the same. Towards the end of November their efforts began to show fruit:

> 25th: Sunday School at 3 p.m. The Windorah coach in at 6 p.m. and we got nine parcels from Miss Duncausin for the Christmas tree. Held our first song service at 7 p.m.

These "song services" were casual affairs and soon there were between a dozen and eighteen attending. What pleased the Sisters was that once folk attended they tended to do so fairly regularly thereafter despite no expectations being put on them. A short sermon only would be given and a sociable chat would follow at the end. These evenings opened the door for many meaningful discussions later on a more personal level during the week, especially with women, but occasionally with men. The fact that there was company and a cup of tea available most hours of the day and early evening, unless the Sisters were very busy, made Brisbane Home a popular venue, even with those just "blowing through". And if the Sisters were busy, it was still possible to sit down, relax and read the books they put out—which they later expanded into a library when their luggage finally arrived.

Excitement mounted as Christmas Eve, the night of the Christmas-tree party, approached:

> 24th: Very busy. Mail in yesterday and such heaps of parcels and books from home. Mr Smith and Mr Williams motored out and brought in a tree for the toys tonight.
>
> We got word at about 4 p.m. that our furniture would arrive in a couple of hours! So we hurried up and after fixing the Christmas tree ready for 8 p.m. we went along to see the camels, 75 in all, slowly wending their way along the flat. They stopped at the hotel and were unloaded for an hour or so, and then they moved along to the hospital where they were unloaded for a good three hours. We were not able to be with them all the time. [She reported later that no sooner was the furniture unloaded than it started to rain, but they had to leave it stacked up outside because of the Christmas party. They had only 5 cm of rain during their time in Birdsville so this situation was ironic.]

> 64 turned up at the Christmas tree! We started at 8.45 p.m. It looked very nice and the wee folk were so excited about it all, not having seen one before. When Santa made his appearance the shouting was loud and we soon distributed the toys and gave Santa three cheers and bade him goodbye... At 10 p.m. the children being tired, and ready for bed, we closed our entertainment. They are all satisfied that it is the best Christmas yet in Birdsville. A beast was killed in the township and Christmas meat distributed.

The killing of a beast was always the occasion for celebrating, especially among the Aborigines. The Sisters never lacked for beef because the cattle drovers and nearby stations were aware of their needs and provided fresh meat regularly.

Water, though, was a problem. The Sisters had to carry their own in buckets from the billabong, until Omadally Musha and his camel train arrived with a tank, but then there was too little rain to fill it. The water shortages were dire at times and the Sisters used leftover tea to wash their hair with. Throughout their whole stay they were limited to half a bucket of water per day for the washing of themselves. They learned of one local family who shared the same small tub of water, one by one, then washed their clothes in it, finally pouring it onto a shrub they hoped to keep alive. Through lack of water there were no fresh vegetables grown locally and only a few wrinkled apples survived the tedious voyage from Adelaide, and then only in the winter. When an Afghan cameleer, Roy Khan, gave Grace a box of apples in appreciation for her dentistry, it was a great treat.

Heatwaves compounded their difficulties. On 17th February 1925, Grace recorded:

> Very hot day. The school had to be closed on account of excessive heat. Temperature 118°. An almost unbearable *hot* northerly wind blowing; the only way to rest is by means of wrapping one's body in a wet sheet. Boyd and I find this a wonderful invention and comply freely with the scheme. The temperature with that raging hot north wind prevented the whole of Birdsville from the slightest rest.

> 21st: Mr Lee returned per car and drove us all down for a dip after tea – it was great. He also sent in a bag of meat but unfortunately the sun smiled on it with vengeance and we had to consign it to the rubbish heap.

Grace believed in sporting activities for health's sake as well as their role in welding a community together. She arranged ping-pong competitions and picnics and swims, and decided a tennis court would be a good addition. She floated the idea and found support for it, so became part of the organising committee and arranged for wire netting to be purchased and sent. She participated in the hard manual work in levelling the ground. Once it was up and running, she arranged many matches on it.

By the time the next Birdsville Races came around, she and Catherine were playing an important role in organising community activities:

> 8th: Children's races this afternoon. I went in for the ladies' race and came 4th. We hurried away at 6 p.m. and Mrs Williams ran us down in the car for a dip. We had Mrs Crabb, Reese and Griffin for tea, all of whom had to give a hand to clear up afterwards as we had arranged a ping-pong tournament to be held in our kitchen. However, we were ready for the players at 8 p.m. and started off—ending in a win for me. Afterwards we had a little music and supper, winding up about midnight. Everybody seemed to enjoy the evening.

In all of this, Grace was espousing Flynn's concept of developing a sense of family in the bush as pivotal to improving the social fabric. With a united and caring community, life in the bush would be much more pleasant for women and children.

But what sort of person was this human dynamo who quietly and sensibly achieved so much? In photographs she looks dignified and rather austere, but remembrances of her were of a warm, pleasant lady with a very positive outlook: "Grace by name and graceful by nature". In private, though, she experienced depression from time to time. Although none would have suspected this, she confided about it in her writings. Inadequate diet may have contributed to this, while another of her trials sprang from the long delay between the mails. Some mails from Windorah were a month late and one was two months late because "it appears the mailman stopped at Beetoota for the races—mail seems to him to be only a secondary consideration". She came from a large and affectionate family and when there was no news for such long periods she wondered if all was well. At such times she suffered severe homesickness. Then when the mail arrived her spirits lifted at once.

During their work, Catherine Boyd was very happy to play the support role to Grace. For example, they had been in Birdsville a whole year before Catherine pulled her first tooth. Younger and less experienced, Birdsville was a seminal phase in her life and later nursing.

As further medicines and equipment arrived, the nurses were able to minister with greater effectiveness within the community. They reversed the effect of sandy blight on the eyesight of dozens of children. A dental chair and anaesthetics were obtained by two enthusiastic supporters in Brisbane who went from dentist to dentist requesting donations, and the efficiency of the dental work in Birdsville took a giant leap forward.

In March 1924, Grace decided to take matters into her own hands regarding the water supply in the town hole, something that had concerned her since their arrival.

> 17th: The river is rising slowly, not into the town hole yet. A dead horse, which is not the most pleasant thing, was at the edge of the water hole. Five of us women burnt it, although the men tell us the flood waters will not reach it. Still, the carcase is in the main channel to the town hole so we prefer to be certain of it.
>
> 18th: The water is running into the town hole, so we are pleased we burnt the horse.

The first baby born in the hospital was Lyle Morton on 21st May 1924. [Lyle was destined to marry an AIM Sister from the Birdsville Hospital, and he and Phyllis (nee Beech) were a great help and support for succeeding generations of nurses there. In the course of time their son Geoff also married an AIM Sister, Bev (nee Frankum). Geoff and Bev have two sons...]

Not all bushmen were as supportive as the Morton family of the work carried out by the Sisters. One old bushman named Long preferred to treat himself for beri-beri. What did he need the hospital for, he asked? He stayed in his camp 19 kilometres away and refused to budge. Grace commented: "Expect he will come in one of these days, but these bushmen are ridiculously averse to women."

Sadly, though, Long had misdiagnosed his own condition. When mates carried him in to Sister Grace he was too far gone from advanced heart disease for her to help him:

> He died at 11 p.m. after a struggle for eight hours. I had to let him have his mattress on the ground; he just begged to have it there, as the wire mattress was too soft for him. These poor old bushmen are so used to the ground for sleeping that they are uncomfortable on a bed. He managed to sign his will before he died. It was a happy release for him from the pain and breathlessness.

There being no morgue, Long was buried the following day because of the heat:

> The funeral took place this morning at 11 a.m. The policeman brought his car and the body was carried in the back; Sister and I were in the front. I read the burial service. Could not procure timber to make a coffin so the body was sewn up in cloth and then in white calico. I have written to his wife who lives in Adelaide.

Grace travelled on errands of mercy when a patient was too ill to be brought into the hospital. In one instance she went 224 kilometres by car to Cordillo Downs to treat a young man, but the spare fuel turned out to be kerosene and they had to walk to the nearest homestead and wait until replacement fuel arrived. Then they struggled over flooded, rough country. After further mishaps, she arrived and treated the injured man successfully.

On the return "our luck was not on that track as only a mile away two tyres were flat. Mr Lee, when jacking up the wheel, broke that implement: and so we were 'jiggered' for tyres. We had to come the remaining 44 miles to the Bluff on three flat ones but we got here, although the covers were badly knocked about. Will have to stay here tonight and drive the buggy in tomorrow. I can never forget the consideration and respect I received from the men en route."

Thus it was that she completed the five-day odyssey by horse and buggy. She did not complain, but pondered how the execution of such arduous mercy missions could be improved. She concluded that John Flynn's planned wireless network and Flying Doctors could provide the only answer. At every opportunity in her letters and later on in talks she gave, she promoted Flynn's vision of a Mantle of Safety.

On 11th August 1925, John Flynn and George Towns arrived in Birdsville to experiment with wireless, and Grace especially was very excited. Flynn was determined that "the dumb bush must speak" to banish its isolation forever. Their experiments in the Inland had aroused great interest already but were not achieving what Flynn had hoped. They lugged in the cumbersome apparatus and set up in the storeroom of the hospital. Grace wrote in her diary: "The men are staying here and we are delighted to have them. Spent the evening talking." This was typical of Flynn, talking into the wee small hours.

Flynn asked to see their records, which showed that they had treated more than 2000 patients within their first 14 months there, without the benefit of a doctor's help or advice. Grace noticed tears in Flynn's eyes that evening as he scanned their impressive records.

Flynn himself had seen many blind people in the outback being led around by a young guide using a stick or spear. Later the great man wrote that he had been especially delighted to realise that the wonderful gift of sight had been given to many children around Birdsville simply by having the nursing home and Sisters there. It was this realisation that had moved him emotionally.

Battery problems made the next two days experimenting with wireless frustrating and unsuccessful. That evening the Mortons drove in from Roseberth and Flynn christened Lyle:

> After this, all retired to the storeroom to hear a concert in Melbourne. We gathered a few of the neighbours and Mr

> Towns gave us a "listening in" treat and it seemed very real. The concert ended in the National Anthem, which also for the moment turned the old storeroom into a concert hall.

This concert programme from Melbourne excited the locals and popularised the concept of wireless. But Flynn wanted to be able to send and receive personal messages, not simply to listen to commercial stations. Then on the 14th August, messages were received from Barcaldine [near Longreach] in central Queensland. This proved the potential of wireless to break the awesome silence of the bush. Flynn also managed to send three telegrams to Adelaide. However, no signal was picked up from Brisbane and Flynn and Towns decided to battle on elsewhere in their great quest:

> 15th: The wireless is being packed and we feel very sad at thoughts of losing our good friends. The men moved off at about 3.30 p.m. and we both felt very sad and lonely. Mr Towns, on his way in to afternoon tea, stopped at the piano in the kitchen and played Auld Lang Syne, which brought a lump to our throats.

The Sisters, though, were drawing to the end of their pioneering service. "It will be good to have a proper bath again," Grace observed, having spent two years sponging down with water from a bucket or having the occasional swim.

When the time came for them to depart they were overwhelmed by the show of affection that was accorded them. "People travelled for many miles over rough country to be at our farewell, and took precautions to arrive in time. From the things they said we knew we had been truly appreciated, and also that the hospital was now accepted fully by the community."

The "bloody missionaries" had been successful at Birdsville and left behind them a legacy of love and healing that prevailed right into the following millennium.

Grace Francis and Catherine Boyd remained close friends after their adventures in Birdsville. The partnership between those two Christian women had been close to ideal and it held firmly until death separated them.

After Birdsville, Grace, with her own family, owned and ran St Mary's Hospital in Maryborough, Queensland. She remained an enthusiastic supporter of Flynn's vision in talks and in newspaper articles, and in personal correspondence encouraged him to persevere. He invited her to return to serve, and because she felt passionately about the need for wireless networks, she returned three years later to help in the setting up of one at Victoria River Downs (VRD) while nursing there from 1931 to 1933.

She nursed at the pretty Wimmera Home, her colleague being Sister Gwen Hurley. While her reputation as an outstanding nurse grew even greater, Grace's primary objective was to help in developing wireless communications. Overcoming many little problems, she helped to form a network with Darwin and Wave Hill. She also presided over the growth of the radio network between VRD and outback properties, considerably easing the burdens of residents in remote areas.

At the conclusion of her term at Victoria River Downs, Grace returned to Maryborough, but thoughts of the Inland were ever with her. Consequently she worked hard for the Queensland Bush Children's Health Scheme, a branch of which was located in Maryborough.

During the Second World War she was appointed Commandant of the Volunteer Aid Detachment in Maryborough, where she trained and directed over 500 volunteers.

Owing to failing health, she and her sisters in 1946 sold their Maryborough Hospital and came to live in Brisbane. From then onwards she was an ardent and active member of the AIM Council for Queensland.

For her services to nursing generally she was in 1950 awarded the decoration of MBE by His Majesty, King George VI.

The Royal Hotel degenerated until later Sisters had to use umbrellas inside during rainstorms. One report read: "We had a mother and family with an umbrella over them and an outpatient whose finger was in a bath with an umbrella over him. Sister and I were running in all directions with things and then we saw the humour of it all, so we put on our hats and coats and had a cup of tea with an umbrella over the tea tray." A new Birdsville

Hospital was imperative and Flynn built it in 1936 to the acclaim of Harry Afford, the Chairman of the Diamantina Shire, who took off his hat at the opening ceremony and declared, "People of Birdsville, this is a bloody miracle. We've got a proper hospital." The stockmen laughed and slapped their sides in agreement. But this new hospital burnt down in 1951. During the inferno, Sisters Mona Henry and Lillian Whitehead barely escaped with their lives and lost all their possessions besides the pyjamas they wore. However, they refused to leave Birdsville and showed the same courage and determination to serve the community that had characterised Grace Francis and Catherine Boyd.

Out of the ashes grew a bigger and better Birdsville hospital, and Grace was delighted to attend its opening in 1953. She was shown the diary she had written all those years previously, it being one of the very few items to survive when the hospital had been destroyed by fire. She was also amazed at how the Sisters had escaped the fire—their lives were saved because the side door that was usually wired up on the outside had been inadvertently left open that night! There would have been no other possible avenue for escaping the flames. It transpired that the policeman had chased crows that very afternoon onto the veranda of the hospital and had unwired the side door to try to catch and destroy them. The crows had been pecking out the eyes of baby goats, infuriating him. Despite the law of the bush that states "leave a gate as you find it", he had neglected to secure the door again. The "Divine hand", Grace wrote, "had moved to save our two Sisters".

Grace was to make one more trip to the Inland. On his last visit to Brisbane, shortly before he died, her friend John Flynn said to her, "Sister, I feel strongly that there ought to be some sort of memorial erected on the site of the old Elsey station homestead. I wonder if you would undertake to see that it is done?" This was to acknowledge the debt he and the Inland owed to Jeanie Gunn and the advice she had given him all those years before.

Flynn died soon after this visit. In loyalty to her leader's memory, Grace set about the task of realising his desire. She was responsible for obtaining the money necessary to cover the cost and she was satisfied only when she learned that the memorial had been erected. But now she desired to see it. So, in collaboration with other friends, a plane was chartered specially for a trip to the Inland. Visits were paid to Birdsville, Alice Springs (where she attended a communion service in the John Flynn Memorial Church), Oodnadatta, and the Elsey Station Memorial. Returning home, she felt at peace, satisfied she had fulfilled the last expressed wish of her dear friend.

Grace was now to face a lengthy illness, but she did so with the courage that characterised her whole life. She passed away on 19th September 1959, in Brisbane, aged 67 years.

Her life had been a model of service to others. She had given of her best to those sick in body, mind and spirit.

In 1963, two cottages were built alongside the Birdsville hospital to accommodate elderly bushmen who needed to spend their final years in retirement in the precincts of the town. It was fitting that the AIM named one of its two cottages the Francis Cottage. Grace would have enjoyed the humour but also understood the sentiment of one old timer who declined a place at Francis Cottage, saying, "No thanks, city life isn't for me."

Flynn was proven correct in handpicking Grace to establish the first AIM hospital at Birdsville because it had been such a difficult and inhospitable challenge. She fulfilled his commission: "A thing done well becomes a tradition that those who come after must follow. And people can always achieve more for themselves than they do. The supreme thing for us is to plant big ideals."

How did other nurses respond to Flynn's high expectations in such earthy and often difficult environments? Let us look at snapshots of some of them.

How the Sisters Were Dressed

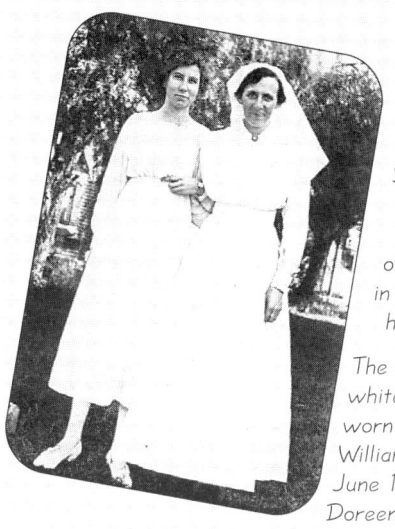

Anti-clockwise from top: Sister Latto Bett - the "Little Angel of the North" - in 1912. Note the high white collar.

The traditional all-white uniform with veil is worn here by Sister Jean Williamson at the Oodnadatta Nursing Home, June 1921. With Jean is her companion, Miss Doreen Brown.

Red epaulettes were later added and nurses still tended to dress formally - even when planting a tree!

Dress codes gradually relaxed at the outposts because of the extreme conditions, though most nurses retained a degree of formal dress while on duty and could be immaculate when the occasion demanded. Sister Nina Walters is dressed for the conditions at Innamincka in 1946.

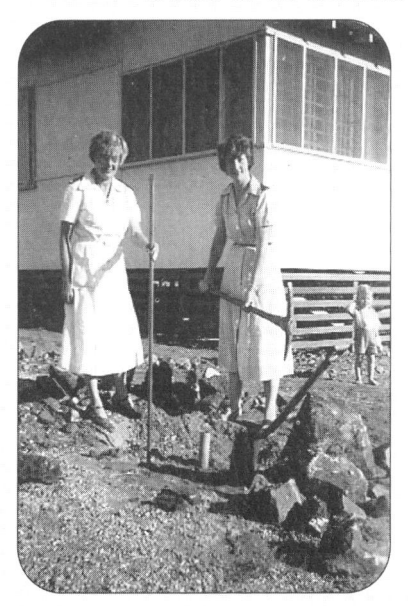

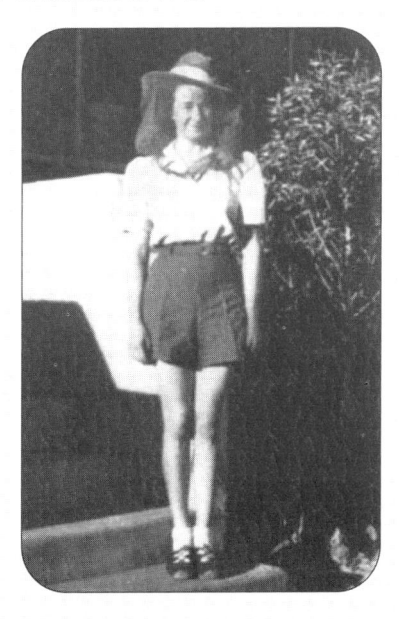

They Also Served

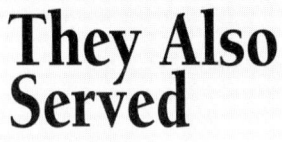

Right: Miss M. Rolland was the very first member of the Melbourne Office Team and served in it for several decades.

Below: Voluntary office teams packed supplies for the nurses and books for their libraries. They also answered correspondence, collected presents for outback children's Christmas parties and in many other ways provided vital logistical support for AIM workers in the field. Beginning in 1915, their unsung, behind-the-scenes service is commendable.

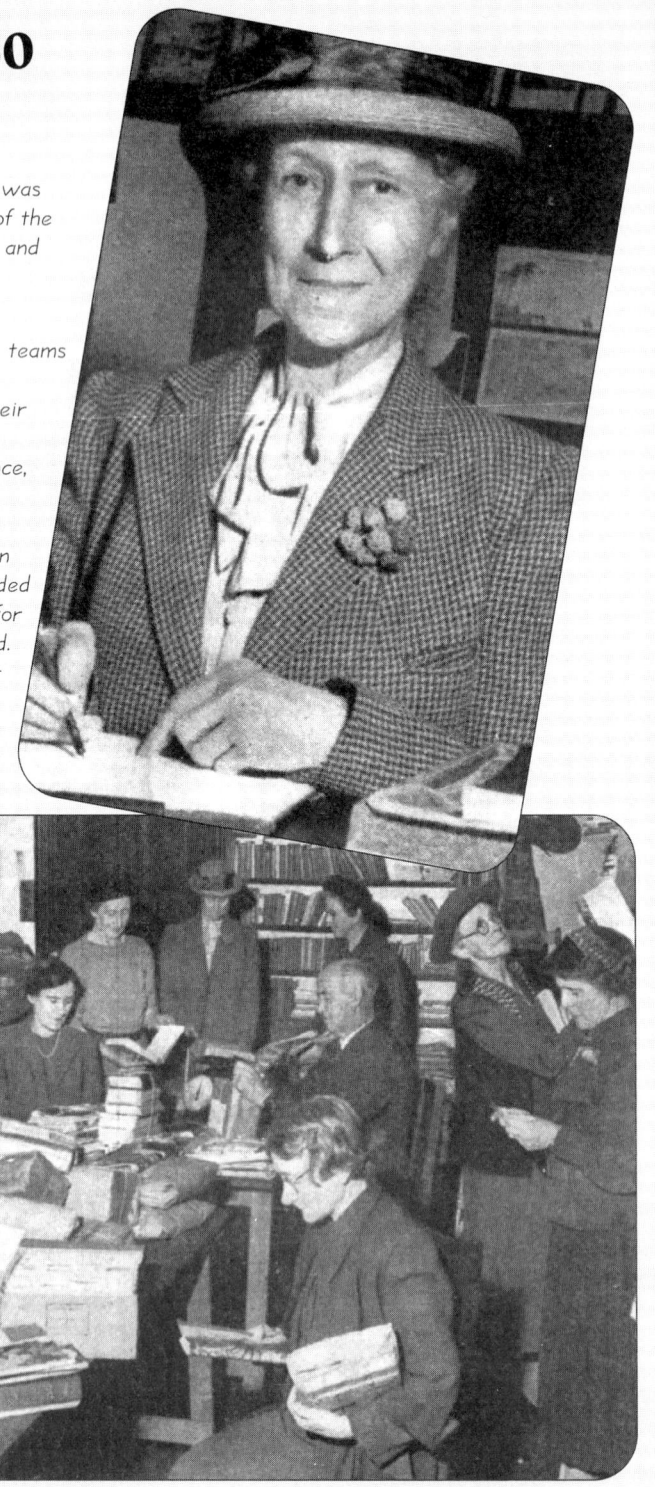

Supplies Came How They Could

Butcher unloading meat – carried in drums and covered by gum leaves – at Halls Creek, WA.

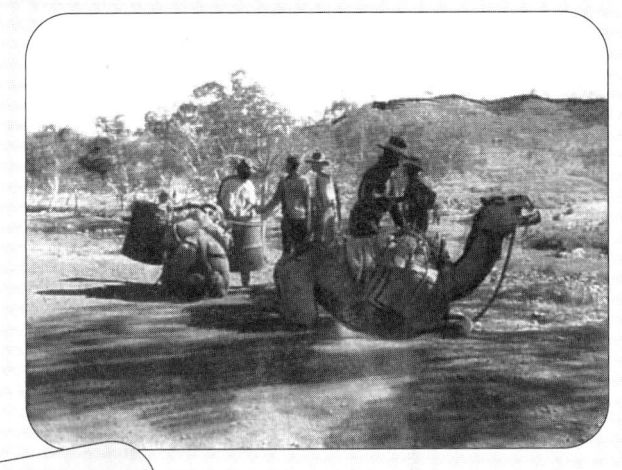

Camel trains brought supplies from the cities to Alice Springs and up the Birdsville Track...

Wagons pulled by animals of all descriptions proved useful...

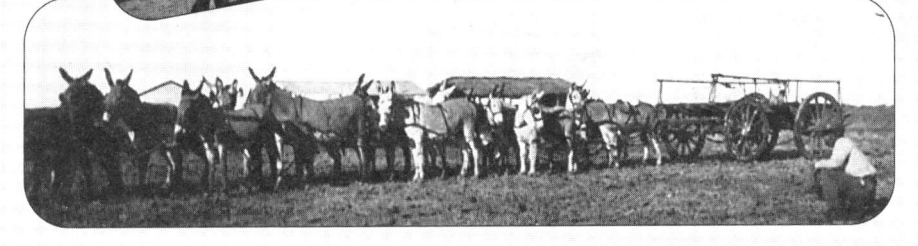

But big trucks were best of all. The legendary Birdsville mailman, Tom Kruse, in 1939. He always got through with the supplies the nurses needed, though seldom on schedule.

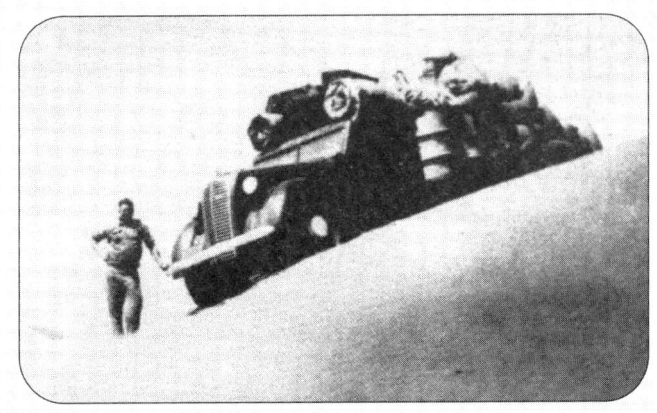

Alternative Transport for Nurses

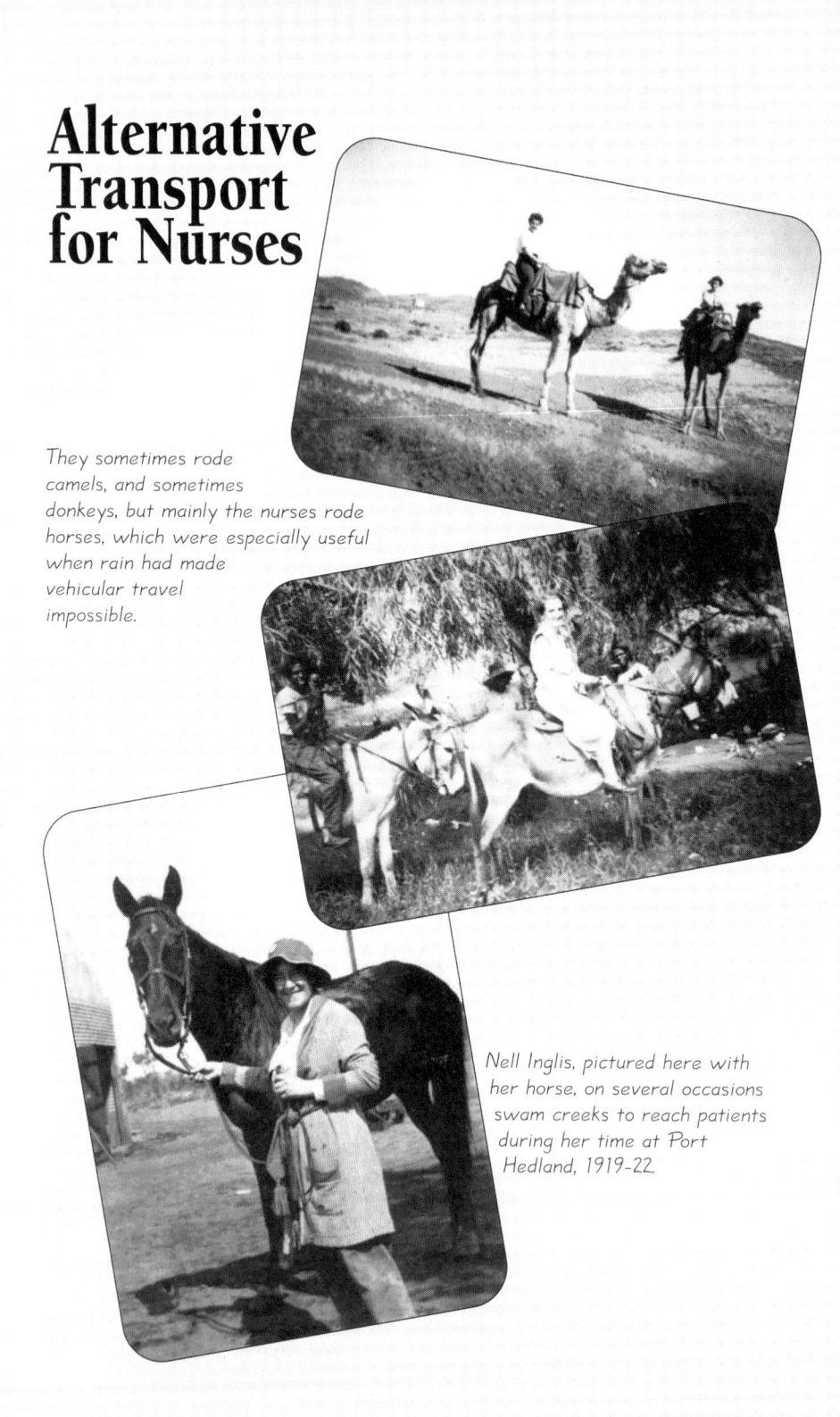

They sometimes rode camels, and sometimes donkeys, but mainly the nurses rode horses, which were especially useful when rain had made vehicular travel impossible.

Nell Inglis, pictured here with her horse, on several occasions swam creeks to reach patients during her time at Port Hedland, 1919-22.

Nurses at Work

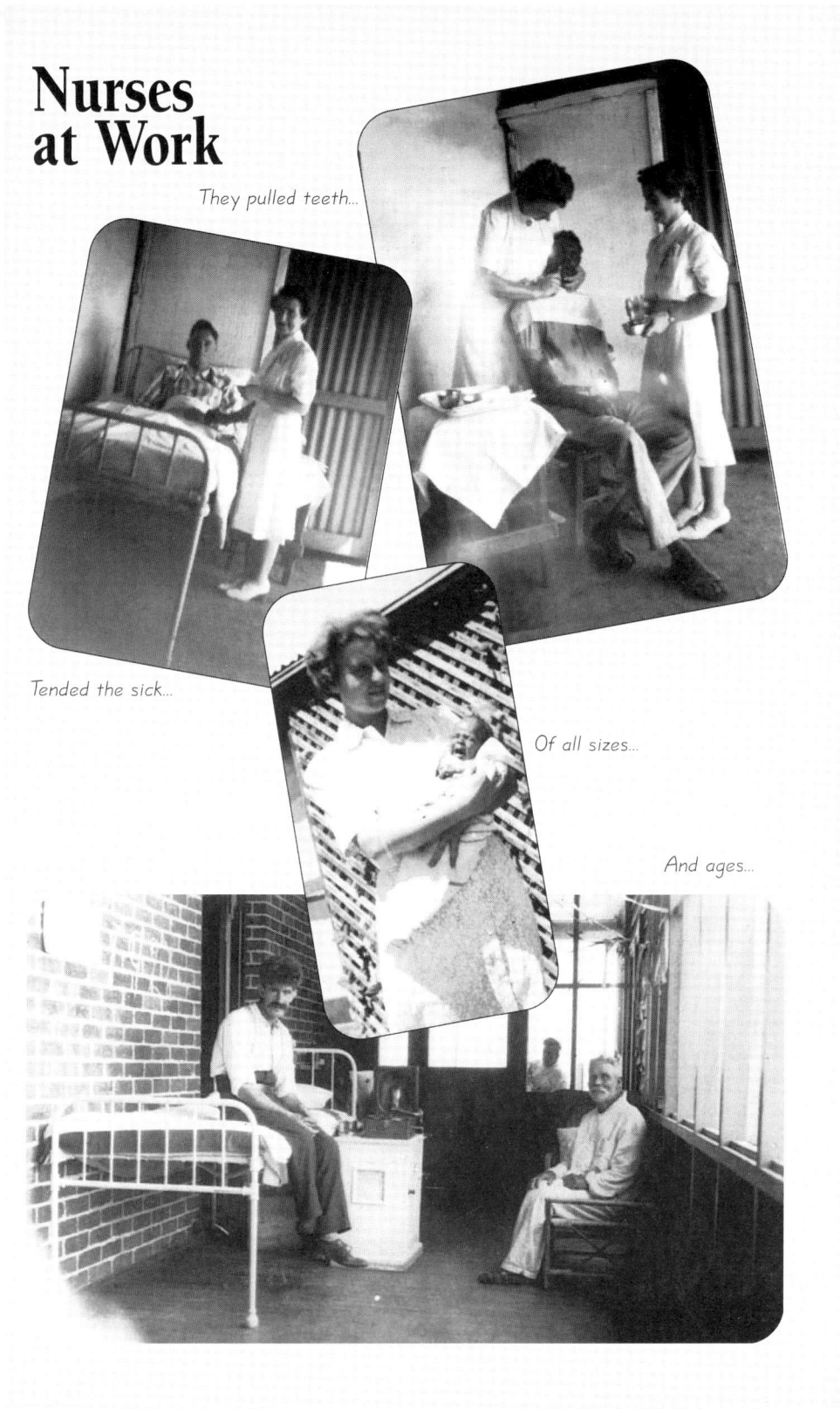

They pulled teeth...

Tended the sick...

Of all sizes...

And ages...

Even if they preferred to sleep outside...

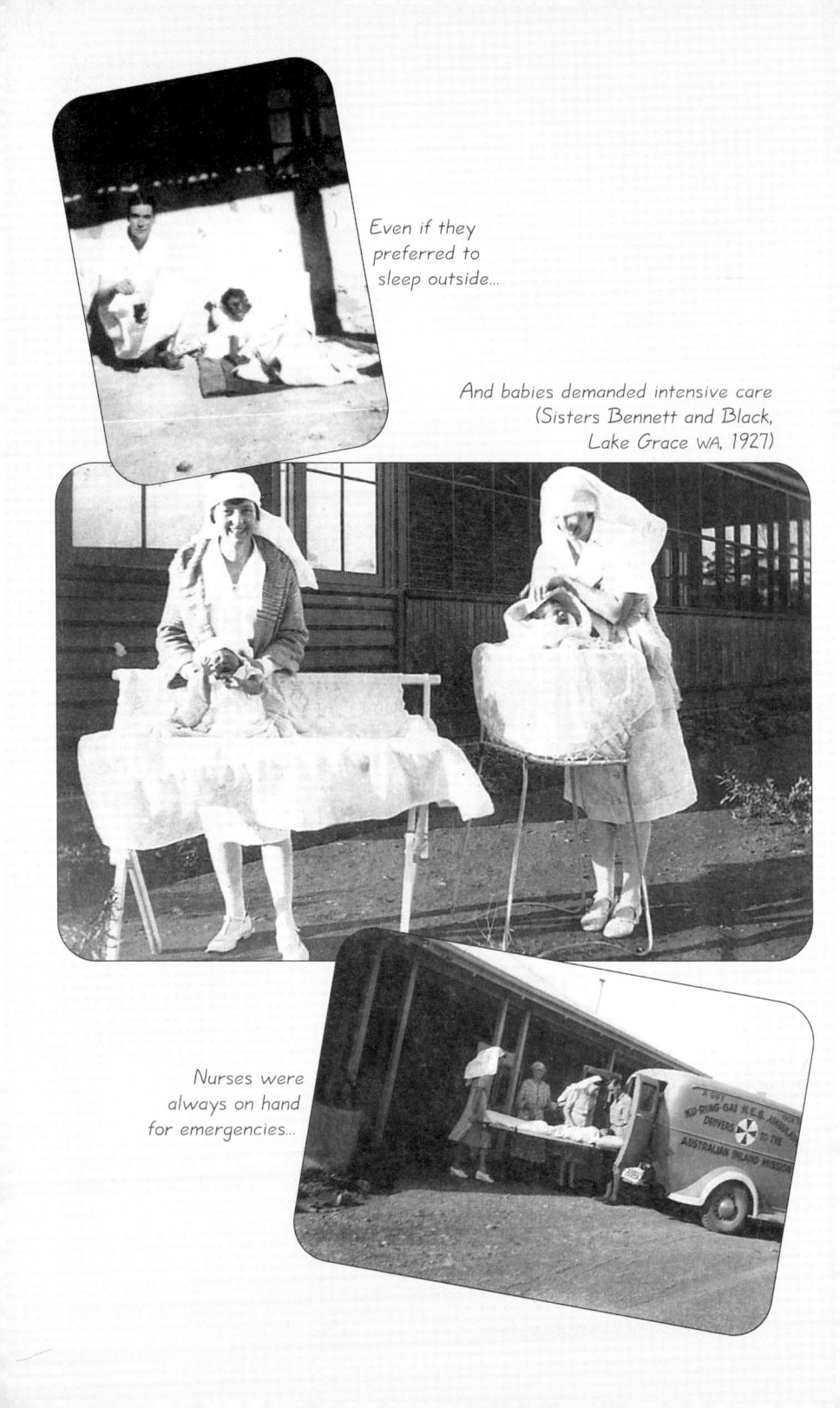

And babies demanded intensive care (Sisters Bennett and Black, Lake Grace WA, 1927)

Nurses were always on hand for emergencies...

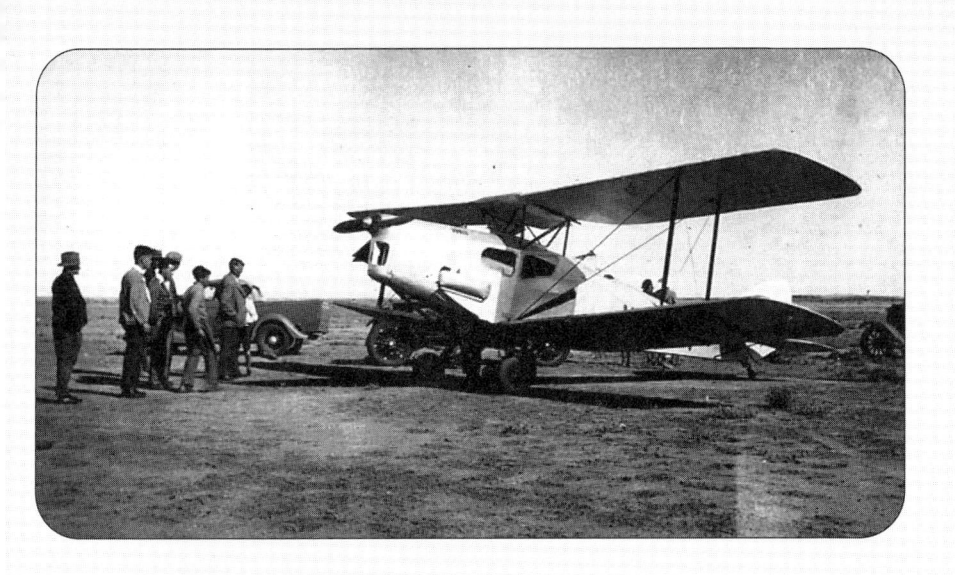

They cooperated with the Flying Doctors on mercy missions (Above: Dragon Rapide aircraft; Pilot Eric Donaldson, Doctor Gordon Alberry)...

tended the sick in Aboriginal camps...

and accompanied patients during emergency evacuations to hospital. In this car (below) Olive Weymouth (nee Bennett) in 1924 took a patient from Halls Creek to Wyndham - a distance of 400 kilometres - for treatment that would save his life.

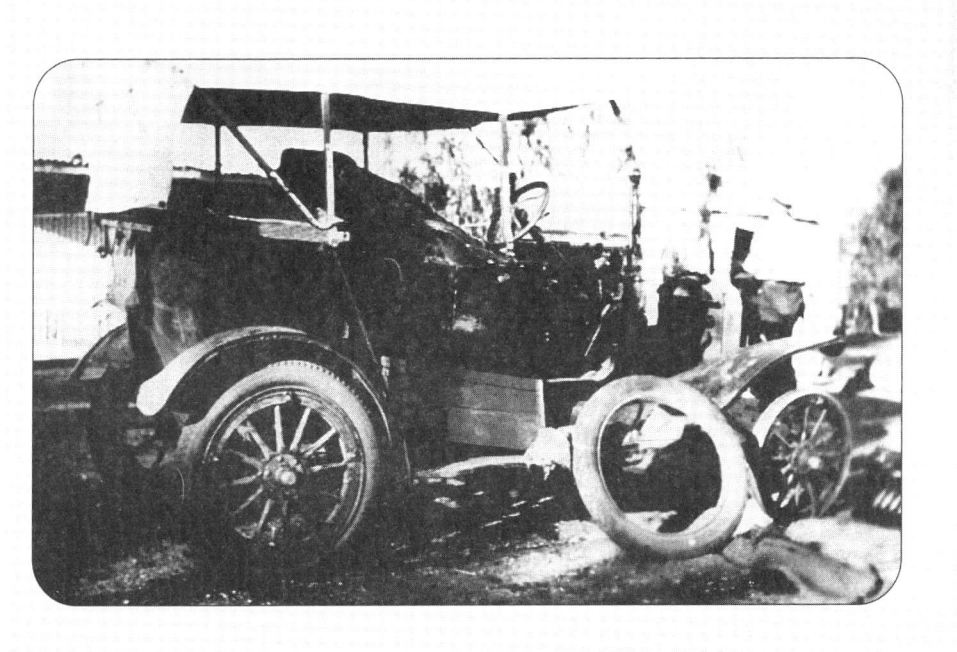

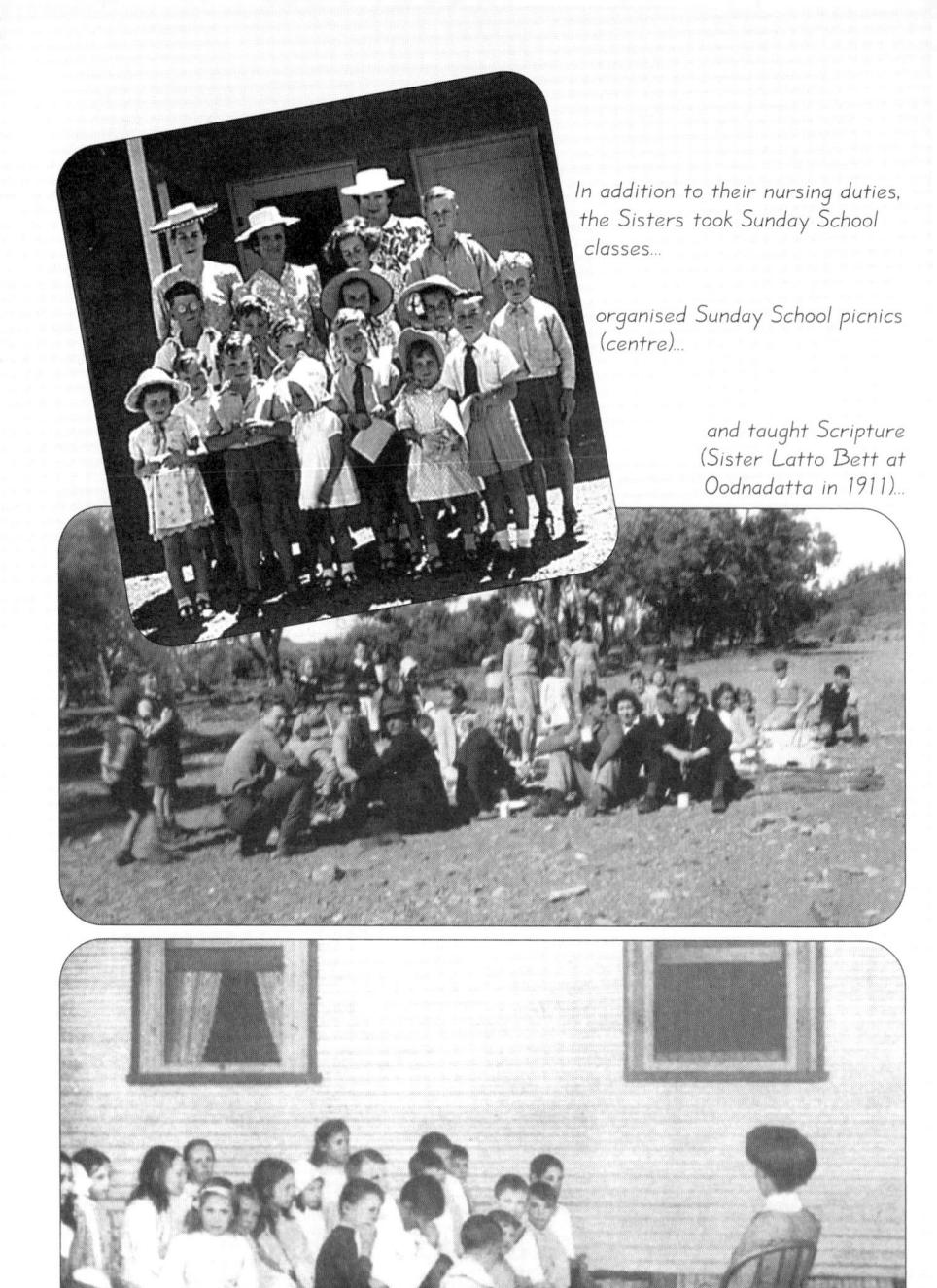

In addition to their nursing duties, the Sisters took Sunday School classes...

organised Sunday School picnics (centre)...

and taught Scripture (Sister Latto Bett at Oodnadatta in 1911)...

7

Flynn's Early Nurses in Snapshot

Flynn's nurses were far more than just nurses, as had always been his intention. From the inception of the AIM in 1912 he intended them to be representatives of Christian love and values in the wider sense. They were to provide friendship and a home from home for men and women in the bush, who may have been away from a caring environment most of their lives. They were to challenge prevailing conditions in the bush socially, spiritually and morally through their own example. Overall, they would illustrate an alternative to the sad lifestyles described in Jessie Litchfield's letter that had first moved Flynn. How far did they succeed in fulfilling this overwhelming challenge? Skipper Partridge, Flynn's longest serving Patrol Padre, observed:

> They are not only "nurses", they are "nurses plus". For if you think of them as just taking their place by the bedside, tending their patient for a specified number of hours, and then being relieved by another mate, you would have the wrong idea altogether. That's why I say they are nurses and something more, and that "something more" may be interpreted on one occasion as a dentist, on another as ambulance officer, on another as social and welfare worker, as a minister, as friend, as confidant or doctor—and a dozen other roles they fill in the lives of the lonely folk of the Inland.

One of these dozen other roles included that of wireless operator. Often tentative when approaching the transceiver itself for the first time, especially in the early days when they needed to transmit in Morse code, the nurses nonetheless felt great relief at being able to consult a doctor at last for difficult cases. And it made their cottage hospitals a communications centre for the townsfolk from which telegrams were sent and received. Furthermore, Flynn's wireless network enabled them to daily communicate with homesteads hundreds of miles away and a social fabric and understanding developed between them and the pioneers that otherwise would have been impossible. Thus the wireless lessened loneliness for the nurses as well as the Inlanders. Rill Gibson, in her first letter home from Innamincka in 1942, wrote: "What fun we have with our transceiver. Today we were talking for 45 minutes and laughing most of the time. Pedalling a la bicycling is necessary when sending a message so that the conversation lasts until the legs get weary." All AIM nurses shared her delight with the social interaction ushered in by the transceiver.

But the transceiver did not substitute entirely for personal interaction and the Sisters sometimes got lonely. Allan Vickers, the renowned Flying Doctor, recalls flying to Birdsville.

> When Eric, my pilot, and I arrived, both Sisters [Campbell and Fanshawe 1930–1932] came out to greet us. But they said not a word. They had never seen us before and here we were, two strange men loaded down with parcels. Eric, with his greying hair and distinguished appearance, looked more like a doctor than I, but they weren't sure which of us was which. When eventually I made the introductions they both began to talk at once. They still hadn't talked themselves out when we left to return to Cloncurry the following day.

Besides the social revolution it caused, wireless rapidly proved its value in saving lives without a rescue mission needing to be flown. For example, in 1931, four-year-old Kevin McCarthy was writhing in pain on the banks of the Cooper Creek. One of his legs had been badly burnt by a spill of billy tea and the wound stretched from his knee to the thigh. It was almost dark by the time Ina Currey and Elizabeth Burchill had crossed the swollen creek to reach him. They gave emergency treatment and by next morning he was resting comfortably in the AIM Nursing Home at Innamincka.

Days later the wound was healing when Kevin developed toxic poisoning and became dangerously ill.

Hurriedly pedalling the newly installed transceiver into action, Elizabeth Burchill tapped out a message in Morse code to the Flying Doctor in Cloncurry, 1140 kilometres away. Across the airwaves came the reply from the doctor. The treatment he advised

EARLY NURSES

saved Kevin's life. Six decades later Kevin affirmed that, "I owe my life to the Sisters and the mission. The nearest doctor was far away and all the nurses had was that pedal wireless." Elizabeth Burchill agrees, "Kevin would never have survived the hazardous drive to the nearest doctor at Tibooburra, 400 kilometres away."

The transceiver also enabled the Sisters to perform minor operations under the instructions of the Flying Doctor hundreds of miles away. At Innamincka, in 1940, Doctor Woods decided not to fly out 300 miles from Broken Hill but to tell the Sister step-by-step how to treat a dislocated shoulder and relayed the instructions:

> DOCTOR: Have you any assistants? Over to you.
> SISTER: Yes; Connell, the policeman, and a stockman. Over to you.
> DOCTOR: All right. Sit the patient in a chair. Over to you.
> SISTER: He is now sitting in a chair. Over to you.
> DOCTOR: Get Connell to hold the patient's elbow close to his side and the stockman to hold the forearm. Are you doing that? Over to you.
> SISTER: Yes. What next? Over to you.
> DOCTOR: Hold the forearm at the wrist in a horizontal position, and then force it outward away from the body until it won't go any further. Over to you.
> SISTER: Oh! The shoulder clicked back into position!

Within minutes the Sister reported that the patient was feeling comfortable and much relieved.

Similar medical procedures relayed by transceiver met with mixed success when conducted by the men outback without the presence of a nurse to monitor progress. For example, the Sisters put the patient in direct communication with the Flying Doctor when a man at Roy Hill station was in agony from a very bad toothache and they were too far away to help themselves. Doctor Allan Vickers then gave instructions over the radio for removal of the offending tooth: they were to fetch a certain size of pliers that would be in the garage and he would direct them how to sterilise the pliers. Since Roy Hill did not have a transceiver, they had

117

asked Balfour Downs to help. So Vickers' instructions were relayed by "fence telephone"—passed from neighbour to neighbour— from Balfour Downs to Roy Hill. He then said the patient should lie down on a large table and have his gums massaged with whisky to act as anaesthetic. He suggested they give the patient a stiff whisky while they were about it. Then he detailed how the tooth was to be removed step by step, all relayed to Roy Hill station by fence telephone.

Apparently the surrogate dentist and spectators all gained moral support from the same bottle of whisky used for the patient. They then opened a second bottle to ensure their nerves were quite strong enough to endure the painful procedure to follow. Finally the dentist set to work.

The operation proved to be a roaring success, excepting for the fact that the wrong tooth was extracted! But such errors were few and far between and no serious mistake in treatment by radio was ever made, mainly because the Flying Doctor's policy was to undertake a medical flight rather than to take a risk.

Numerous unanticipated advantages grew out of Flynn's wireless network for the nurses besides the direct medical ministry. For example, nurses often had trouble with bushmen who refused to do what the nurse instructed—partly because they "knew better than a woman" and partly because they were genuinely tough, for example discounting bed rest for broken ribs unless it was accompanied by the spitting out of blood. But when wireless arrived, the nurses discovered they could get a doctor's instructions which carried a lot more weight than their own. And it was more than just a "male thing" because the bushmen held the wireless in some kind of awe. The Sisters discovered with delight that their patients would obey whatever the wireless told them to do, and it was left to the Sisters to interpret exactly what the message had said—or even what it might have meant to say if expanded upon. Doctor Allan Vickers noted: "You can bully a bushman quite well over the radio!"

Indeed, especially in the early days, the wireless was believed implicitly by some of the Inlanders. There was a story Skipper Partridge would tell to new Sisters to give them insight into the awe in which it was held. It seems that a certain homestead wanted to send their wireless set back to the AIM because it "made all the clocks wrong" and they were going to lose their hired hand who was sick of meals being served at odd times. On investigation Skipper discovered how this complaint had arisen. The listeners all believed the radio implicitly, so when it gave the time they changed the watches and clocks in the immediate vicinity, leaving others elsewhere alone. But they had been listening on short wave to the BBC and other overseas stations, so the times given were hopelessly out for Australia. Their conclusion was that the radio mysteriously changed the time on their clocks. Skipper's explanation placated the hired hand, who reversed his decision to leave.

Another role Flynn's nurses had to fulfil was that of a pharmacist. Sister Allen (Wimmera Home 1937–39) explains:

> Now with regard to medicines, we had to do our own dispensing. We had our little scales that we measured everything up with, but we were rather nervous to begin with. My friend and I always saw to it that we took a dose of our own medicine because we felt that if we poisoned anyone we'd rather be dead than face the consequences.

Furthermore, the nurses had to be diagnosticians; at least until the radio network was operating. And many unusual cases presented themselves, as in the case of a baby whose vomiting threatened his life. Sister Langham (Wimmera House 1935-37) solved baby John William's vomiting and loss of weight—it was the goat's milk.

> Goats eat anything this time of the year, causing the milk to be bitter and upset the baby. We tried him on milk from our hospital cow and he tolerated it quite well, but after one day it rained and the cows went bush. Result—no milk. However, there was a plentiful supply of Nestlés [powdered milk] in the store. We commenced with it and baby went straight ahead.

Also, unlike nurses in city hospitals, Flynn's angels had to cook and launder for patients and undertake the cleaning and upkeep of the hospital itself. Food was often scarce and very different to what they were used to and therefore preparing edible, nutritious meals for the sick was a challenge. Flynn instructed his Patrol Padres to help with maintenance work whenever they were in the vicinity and good working relationships developed between them and the girls, but months might pass before the itinerant minister returned and the Sisters had to fix a lot of things themselves.

These differences in a nurse's daily life between city and country can be glimpsed in their letters home. Here is an extract from one written by Rill Gibson. She and Barbara Clipsham served at Innamincka (1942–43).

> Can I milk goats? Yes, verily, quite expert. We have over a hundred goats but milk about twelve only (quite enough). There is Killarney Kate, Rabbit, Hysteria, Wysteria, Prairie Flower and other equally suitable names for goats. These goats also supply meat. "Jack the Ripper" is an Aborigine and very obliging, so when Sister Blanch requested the brains of the goat he killed, he presented us with the whole head—eyes and all—to mind until morning. On the morrow, under Sister Blanch's and my watchful eye, he gouged out the brains. I declined brains for breakfast, do you blame me?... As you know, we take it in turns to be nurse and cook, week and week about. "Nurse" milks goats, attends to wireless sessions, does all the housework and garden including Monday morning's washing, to say nothing of acting in the official capacity of Florence Nightingale. We also teach school during the day. "Cook" cooks. I am "cook" from tomorrow and my troubles (and everyone else's) begin in earnest.

The Aboriginal culture was a bit of a shock to most of the young nurses when they arrived from the city, as it had been with Rill watching the brains being gouged out of the goat's head described above, but they soon became fond of the friendly Aborigines despite the differences. Their diaries and letters are sprinkled with interesting anecdotal material, including Sister Janet Hepburn's (Maranboy 1917–18) description of an Aboriginal servant who sported a top hat swathed in a large red handkerchief:

> Miss Gillespie, desiring that his manner should equal his headgear in splendour, instructed him in the art of lifting his

hat in greeting and farewell; and this he did in most courtly style until one luckless day when he thus revealed four slices of bread and butter he was carrying home to his wife in this convenient receptacle.

Sister Jean Herd (Maranboy 1920–22) made the following observations about Aborigines:

> Friends sent us a small gramophone and some records. These were a great joy to us, but I think an even greater joy to the Aborigines who would stand around the hospital, laughing until the tears rolled down their faces at our music.

Later on she found Aboriginal intervention very helpful:

> Sipping our afternoon tea one afternoon, we saw Paddy [an Aboriginel become very excited. He told us there was a snake under our table. We moved away very quickly; he grabbed it, whirled it around his head until its head flew off. We saw him later, proudly bearing it back to his camp where he ate it.

Yet, as patients, the nurses found Aborigines to be very frustrating. They could withstand great pain without complaint, but seldom wanted to remain inside the hospital building for any length of time, especially if they knew some patient had died there previously. So they would camp outside huddled around their fires, accompanied by relatives—scarcely the best conditions to recover from illness. And again, they would often take off long before their treatment was completed. For infectious diseases, this generated further problems. However, despite these difficulties, the nurses and their Aboriginal patients generally got on well. Here are some observations about specific patients seen with a tolerant eye, beginning with "Rill" Gibson describing a novel approach to diagnosis practised by the same Jack the Ripper she mentioned in her previous letter:

> He told us that Annie, his missus, was "very sick". He had stood her up and she fell down. So he stood her up again, and she fell down again. He stood her up for the third time, but she fell down again. He concluded she was really sick. I thought I would find her unconscious or even dead.

In fact Annie was conscious but very ill, so Rill transferred her to the Hostel to receive proper care. But Annie returned home soon afterwards because she was missing her fire.

The pain threshold of Aborigines was legendary. The Sisters at Alice Springs roped in the visiting Doctor Walker to help in the case of Toby, an Aboriginal warder who had been attacked by his prisoners while having a snooze two miles outside the town. The doctor reported:

> The prisoners attacked him with their axe and chopped his skull open, partly gouged out his right eye and made a large gash in his neck through which the carotid artery could be seen beating. They left him for dead and escaped. However, in a few hours he regained consciousness, to find his forehead hanging over his cheek. He picked it up and tucked it under his hat and walked in the two miles to the hostel. Here I spent two and a half hours picking out splinters of bone, eyebrows, eyelashes, pieces of dirt; then cleaned it up with iodine and carbolic and put in 16 stitches without anaesthetic. He did not flinch—so remarkable is the Aborigines' endurance and ability to bear pain. Meanwhile, a mile away, I could hear the whole camp singing a death wail. However to my surprise, and everyone else's, he recovered!

Ina Currey (Innamincka 1930–31) records a fairly typical interaction between the cultures:

> Billy was brought in to us with a poisoned arm – and a general septicaemia temperature of 105 degrees. There has been a big corroboree in Innamincka; Billy said, "Perhaps sumping bin bite him,": but something *didn't* bite him, our diagnosis was that Billy had cut into his veins to get blood to stick on his cockatoo feathers, and then smeared himself all over with red ochre, which got into the nicks on his arm.
>
> I paid him a late visit that night, made him comfortable, and gave him a drink.
>
> On going down at 6.30 a.m. I find—Billy had waited to see us away, and then crept back to the corroboree and danced, sick as he was, all night. They got worked up into their usual frenzy and finished with a fight. Billy now has,

in addition to his poisoned arm, a fractured left wrist and a right dislocated shoulder. We thought his 'party' was going to cost him his life last week, but it is quite a cheerful Billy who is now resting contentedly in the police cell. With his arm in splints and his shoulder strapped, he thinks it is a great joke when the Sisters feed him! [With both arms immobilised he could not feed himself.]

And was Ina frustrated by all this and did she want to pack up and leave to return to civilisation? Not a bit of it. A striking characteristic of Flynn's nurses was how positive they remained throughout, despite discomforts and difficulties. Ina loved her nursing at Innamincka so much that she enthused in a letter to Flynn: "Sister Burchill and I have just remembered it is twelve months today since we landed in Innamincka—twelve happy, wonderful months—fancy only twelve more little, short, hurrying months to have of Innamincka—it doesn't bear thinking of!" But unfortunately the enthusiastic Ina fell ill and had to leave early. Later on, though, she married the local policeman, described by Dame Elizabeth Burchill as "the answer to any maiden's prayer", so all ended very happily for one outstanding angel.

It was not only the Aborigines that Flynn's nurses had difficulties with. Most nurses had grown up in a city environment and their interaction with rough, tough individualists such as they encountered in the bush had usually been very limited. So they were launched on a steep learning curve about their new patients and culture from the moment they arrived. In fact a favourite pastime of the men was, "educating the new Sisters". Sister Alice Anderson (Birdsville, 1936–38) recalls:

> We were taught a new language. A large number of anything is a mob—"mobs of flowers, mobs of people and mobs of good luck". Stockmen are called "ringers" while "cowboys" were at a lower level and did the milking and other odd jobs around the place. "Poddy dodgers" and "claypan buccaneers" were men who tried to find "clean skin" cattle and put their own brand on them regardless of the brand carried by the mother. And if you were visiting a neighbour and he was slaughtering, you kept away from his yard

because it would most likely be one of your beasts he was killing, but as you had most likely killed one of his last week it generally evened the score.

Some of the bushies were painfully shy, "Shirtless Charlie" being an example described by Jean Herd (Maranboy, 1920–22):

> Shirtless Charlie had not spoken to a white woman for years. He fled if he saw one of the six or seven women living there. He had been painting the kitchen when Sister arrived in Maranboy earlier than expected, and hid behind the kitchen dresser and fled without meeting her. He stayed away at his mine until six months later when he was carried in unconscious with malaria. He recovered and it was hard to keep him away after that.

Other bushmen were very "macho" and would not heed nursing advice. Olive Weymouth (nee Bennett; Hall's Creek, 1923–25) wrote:

> Bob Smith was opening a bottle of lemonade when it exploded and a portion of glass struck his radial artery. Of course, blood flowed everywhere. He walked up to us and we applied a tourniquet and I put a few stitches in the wound and put him to bed with his arm elevated. We urged him to go to the nearest doctor in Wyndham, but he thought that it didn't look like much so he didn't go—it wasn't a very inviting journey. We tried to point out to him the danger of this bursting at any time and his bleeding to death. Still no response; men can be so obstinate!
>
> Time passed. Then one night we were having a concert in the ward and Bob and another were singing When You and I Were Young, Maggie, when suddenly among all the gaiety a voice cried, "Oh look, Mum, Bob's arm!" There, on the floor, was a pool of blood. The obvious had happened. Fortunately for Bob, we were right there where we could help him. So this was it! It was my turn to accompany a patient to the doctor, so I packed a few necessities and off we went.

It took four days and a difficult journey, with the Wet threatening all the time, before Bob was finally handed over by Olive to the doctor. But his life, which had hung in the balance for a while, was saved.

Another problem the nurses struggled with was drunken patients. With so little healthy entertainment in the bush, some men drank to excess and their health suffered. Skin complaints that would not heal, liver disease, malnutrition and accidents resulted. Sister Anness Calderwood kept a diary in which she described her life while nursing at Oodnadatta (1927–29) and Beltana (1930). The entry for May 4th 1930 reads:

> At 9 p.m. a neighbour called to say there was a man run over on the railway line. They brought him in later and he died at 11 p.m. He had been drinking (had a broken tumbler in his pocket) and had gone to sleep lying across the line. He was the dirtiest white man I have ever seen and the smell was just horrific. They have taken the corpse to the police station. It was a busy morning, cleaning up after the dead man.

Further investigation revealed an ironic twist. The patient's name was Leslie Rooks. He had been sent by railmen to collect beer for them and had then helped them to drink it. Totally drunk, on the way home, Leslie had decided to lie down and sleep, choosing the railway line to snooze on. It was those same railmen he had only just finished drinking with who ran over Leslie and killed him.

Anness Calderwood was an outstanding nurse, driven by compassion. Years after her service with the AIM, while living at Tumby Bay, South Australia, she heard a man who had fallen off the jetty screaming for help. Clad only in thin pyjamas, she rushed out to try and save his life and dived off the jetty into the black sea. The local newspaper recorded:

> This young and splendid specimen of womanhood undoubtedly saved a life, and did so under ugly circumstances. It was dark, the water icy cold, and she knew not the man; who might have been powerful enough to strangle her in the water, as many a rescuer has been by a drowning person. With a total disregard for self, she dared that which, if matched on the field of battle, would probably have been rewarded with a piece of bronze marked "For Valour".

Indeed, as Captain Beth Garrett, herself decorated for valour while a pilot in the RFDS observed (her story will be found in Volume II), the nurses were deserving of far more accolades for bravery than they ever received. Not that they thought so or sought the limelight, but many grateful men and women in the bush knew just how heroic they truly were.

So we see that Flynn chose his nurses carefully because they were required to be so much more than just nurses. In fact, the term "nurse" hardly described their multi-faceted and difficult role at all. Yet hundreds eventually responded to the daunting challenges. And how did Flynn inculcate such high ideals and extraordinary devotion in his nurses? This remains a mystery, but we turn next to his drawing and mentoring of a fine young nurse, Nell Inglis, to provide us with a glimmer of insight.

8

Flynn's Friends—The Inglis Sisters

Flynn, writing to say "farewell" to his Beltana parishioners, in the *Outback Battler* of October 1912, stated:

> I do regret that close touch with you all will be practically ended. If I can read the signs of the times aright, there will now be for me no close touch with anything but the road!

So right from the start, before the AIM had begun its nation-wide ministry, the visionary could see his own future clearly. There would be neither time nor opportunity to form deep friendships; he would be on the road too much.

Indeed, an article I read suggested Flynn was friendless and did what he did in an effort to gain favour with fellow humans. I asked Fred McKay, his friend and successor, to comment on this opinion.

"John Flynn has been described as friendless," Fred told me, "but that's not true. He had many friends, but few close ones because he was never with anyone long enough. All the same, I think that Barber, Simpson and the Inglis sisters, and also his wife Jean, could be considered close friends of his."

Now, I had researched the others Fred mentioned, but knew virtually nothing about the Inglis sisters, apart from the fact that they were AIM nurses. Flynn had sent out hundreds of nurses, most of whom served just two years and then continued with their lives elsewhere. Why were the Inglis sisters different? I made a mental note to follow that one through some time.

Several years later Clive and Margaret Morey put me in touch with Jean Whimp, the daughter of Nell Inglis. Would the mystery be solved at last? Jean kindly supplied me with a large amount of information and documentation, and as I waded through it, understanding began to dawn.

The story began in 1911, before the AIM was even conceived. Nell initiated contact with Flynn when she was still a schoolgirl at

Port Adelaide and he was working around Beltana for the Smith of Dunesk Mission. She had read about Flynn's "Mailbag League", where city folk wrote letters to Inlanders to help ease their isolation and loneliness. However, the Mailbag League had been promoted as being for adults. She wanted to write to children, so wrote to ask permission. Furthermore, she had roped in two of her friends to help, Marion Gillies and Dot McColl (later Hendry), to form a "Triple Alliance".

Flynn was delighted with their intentions, but his reply was typically careful and sensitive. Might not city children be snobbish towards unsophisticated bush kids? And were they to meet one day, what if the city children rejected their country cousins? So he wrote:

> The Manse
> Beltana.
> 20/4/11.
>
> Dear Miss Inglis,
> I was very glad indeed to get your letter today. That article was inadequate. We already are pairing the "daughter" as well. Guess they will do more writing than the mothers anyway…
> I might just add this. Possibly the girls you are paired with—don't know who they may be yet—will be visiting Adelaide later on, and then they will naturally look to you town girls for a little companionship during their stay. There may be some differences in tastes and social standing. Please see that your friends will never let this ever affect them. As Mrs Aeneas Gunn—the well-known Australian writer—put it to me, we want a friendship "that can stand the test of all things".
> I am not anticipating any awkward times ahead at all. I feel sure that any girl who will write will be a good companion, and the girls about here—out of poor homes some of them—are a credit to the place, I think. In the North there is a good deal of almost poverty in the towns. Outside on the runs it is different. But we take all girls who wish, quite irrespective of worldly status, and all joining in at your end must be true to that spirit.

> I would be glad if you would introduce yourself if you happen to get an opportunity at Assembly.
> Thanking you and your friends for writing, and trusting that you will eventually get and give much benefit.
> Sincerely yours,
> J. Flynn.

Nell, acting as the secretary of the Triple Alliance, replied to Flynn's letter enthusiastically. This led to further correspondence. These letters provide an invaluable insight into Flynn's personal nature, and his mentoring of a young girl, so I will quote from them extensively.

By the end of 1911 we read in Flynn's letter regarding "Alice", Nell's penfriend at Beltana:

> Dear Miss Inglis,
> I am so glad that you have found Alice "the splendid girl" I felt sure she would prove. I am little in Beltana, and Alice is very reserved—and shy into the bargain, I think—but it is not difficult to see that there is a deep nature there...

Flynn then explained the problems that were in Alice's home, including poverty. He continued:

> I mention this because I know that you will never breach it to anyone... She must feel the bitterness of her bare home very keenly, and her refined bearing only glows the brighter under the circumstances.

By sharing confidences, Flynn was moving their correspondence to a level of friendship:

> A man cannot help a girl much when he's single. He can only help one girl then. If I devoted enough attention to Alice to get to understand her, people would begin to talk. It's a dead funny world! So you see, I am expecting you to do my work for me.

Flynn then began to school her, perhaps unconsciously, in his own philosophies. She had expressed the desire to raise money to buy furniture for the nursing home at Oodnadatta, so he encouraged her to get started:

> It is always safe to go ahead even if you only have the idea of "something". For instance, the people of Hergott had been talking about the need of a nurse. I urged them to raise money. They all objected to move without a definite scheme... Anyhow last Friday they had a fete, and between that and subs they have sixty pounds. They are struck dumb. It has opened their eyes. Now they can talk and make the Government listen to them, or if the Government won't they can go elsewhere. Sixty pounds is a wonderful thing to open ears.

He then told her that whatever was donated for the new nursing home at Oodnadatta should be in the best taste, because:

> Never let people say "Good enough for the Bush!" The bush must be treated with as much respect as the city, and the people coming from away back need all the love, and all the nice things which can speak of love, that we can give them.

Now he began to nudge her towards serving Christ as a protégé of his.

> By the way, if I may ask, what are your plans for life?... I ask it because we need some of God's best women in the Bush as nurses and deaconesses, and we need many in the city, and shiploads in foreign parts. And I think you have the makings of a good worker. Perhaps you will be surprised at me saying such a thing, but it is true, anyhow. It is a long, dreary, difficult path to take in some respects, but it is interesting, noble and satisfying in others. Perhaps I have said enough. But Australia wants gentle, devoted women to take up Christ's work, and if you are free, and would like to help, I would be glad to hear.

Did Nell want to serve Christ? She recalls: "I can remember playing church with the boys and Nance. We had a huge mangle and used it as the pulpit." But what would she have to offer in the way of Christian service? After a great deal of personal analysis, she decided compassion and serving others were her main character traits. And the more she tussled with the issues, the clearer it became that she was suited to nursing.

She eventually wrote and told Flynn of her decision to become a nurse and to serve God in that capacity, perhaps even in the AIM. Some correspondence is missing because Nell referred to it in an article she wrote, which appeared in *Airdoctor*, issue 136:

> He wrote to me and told me that a girl was coming down to Semaphore who was in trouble with her step-mother and had come to stay with her grandmother to go to school there. He thought she might be terribly lonely and asked me to look her up. So I went down and she was living at Semaphore Park and I invited her up to tea one night. I had younger sisters and we used to see her regularly; yet she said she had never met Mr Flynn. You could see in the letters he wrote how much he cared for people.

Even though he had not met the stepdaughter, Flynn was already "taking care" of her, just as he would care later on for thousands whom he never met.

In the next letter we have, dated 20th March 1912, Flynn is thanking Nell for visiting Dora for him. Dora was the stepdaughter who'd had serious ructions with her stepmother. "Friends and relations are awfully bad property at times," Flynn concluded. He also sought Nell's advice about the pairing of penfriends.

His next letter, the following month, explained his plans for nurses and the part they could play in the outback. This was grooming Nell for her role.

Their friendly correspondence continued and all the time Flynn was inculcating in her his personal philosophies.

Then tragedy struck to divert Nell's plans. Nell had always loved her kindly father who was a sailor, a captain, and the children used to hoist the Adelaide Steamship flag on the flagpole by the shed when they knew he was due home. But he drowned in January of 1913, to the family's great distress. Nell then went out to work as a pupil teacher, as had Flynn himself years before, because she was the eldest child and her mother and five younger children needed all the monetary support she could bring in. Her dreams of training to be a nurse and serve in the AIM had to be put on hold, at least until the family's situation improved. Flynn encouraged her to adopt a positive attitude to the sorrow, disappointment and delay, saying in his letter of 25th June 1913:

> We have to learn lessons in patience. If you are reserved for work away Inland you will need all the teaching you get. The isolated life is very trying at times, but those who have had trials of waiting, and sorrow, and have learned the secret of joy independent of all outward circumstance, will easily bear the isolation and have a bit of pluck to communicate to others into the bargain... the chief value is so that we can help others. Those who have disciplined and subdued the ardent desires and passions of the heart, and patiently borne disappointment in the 20–30 stage, seldom suffer much afterwards. "The same old thing" is passed by lightly and new joys are easily cultivated. And when one has to stand by and help a younger sufferer, the memory of our own warfare makes us kinder and more intelligent in sympathy.
>
> I am glad that Dora is doing well. Give her my kind regards, please, when next you meet her....
>
> Meanwhile I hope that you will have strength and grace to go on to perfection.
>
> > With kind regards,
> > Sincerely yours,
> > J.Flynn.

Flynn was no hypocrite as a mentor. Everything he advised young Nell was lived out in his own life. As an example of his patience, consider that he published in the *Inlander* of October 1919 a visionary article about the potential of wireless, pilots and Flying Doctors to combine to save lives in the bush—and used Nell's term of Triple Alliance as title to the article—but it was a difficult and discouraging decade before his own Triple Alliance became an accepted reality.

In a further letter to Nell in 1913, Flynn wanted to publish in church newspapers that she was intending to serve as a nurse in the AIM "if the way continues open". He was anxious to parade candidates in the media in an effort to drum up support and encourage others to join. He had a manpower crisis at the time that threatened to worsen with the approach of war. She agreed to her intentions being published.

Little by little, step-by-step, Flynn had led the young girl into his missionary work. To an outsider it might seem that Flynn had spent a lot of effort on just one lass but the dividends would prove to be tremendous. Furthermore, the process he used tells us so much about the man and gives insight why it was that many fine women served him so loyally over so many years.

Nell remained faithful to her commitment to serve in the Inland. She was able to enter training to become a nurse in 1915, aged 22. During that same year she received a card to tell her that her boyfriend had been killed in battle. She struggled with her tragic loss but set her heart to do well in her chosen career. "I could not imagine myself working in an office just earning money all my life. I wanted to do something worthwhile."

She completed her training with honours in 1918, winning a gold medal. She then did a further six months at the Melbourne Women's Hospital to get midwifery. This was at Flynn's insistence.

There it was that she made good friends with brave Sister Janet Hepburn, who had launched the AIM nursing home in Maranboy (1917–18) and told Nell what to expect:

> I sent Flynn a letter full of the problems I found there, especially working without having a doctor nearer than Darwin to refer to and the attitude of some of the men, who told us that "women only bring trouble". He answered my list of complaints carefully point by point and gave me great encouragement, but then he'd torn off a scrap of paper and popped it in with his letter. On it he wrote "Look up! Buck up! Shut up!" I took more notice of those words than the rest of his reply. And he was right, you know. As I approached the problems with a positive faith, doing my best, it all worked out—including some very tricky medical cases. Soon the men had accepted us, would do anything for us, and the hospital became the social centre. And they would take books away by the sack full and were very grateful that we could give them reading material; until then, all they'd had to read, they told us,

were the labels on jam tins. But for me, Flynn had given me an approach to life that works, by telling me to "Look up! Buck up! Shut up!"

Flynn also continued to mentor Nell and wrote an encouraging letter towards the end of 1918 in reply to Nell's feelings of inadequacy and her difficulties with the Matron there.

> I understand that the Matron at Melbourne Women's is not the most genial that ever adorned a Hospital, but the girls with sense get along alright. I don't think I would like to be a Matron. Have heard of several not loved to point of rapture... You won't fail! Pity there isn't another medal to win.

He then tackled her upcoming service for the AIM:

> You must not worry about the future. Your life will unfold as you go along. One of the great things is to know your limitations, and keep on working just a little <u>beyond</u> them. That's how you push them further and further out. And it is well to remember that comparatively little teaching is done <u>by word</u>, and that comparatively small results are obtained by <u>conscious</u> effort in spiritual things. The silent lives often accomplish more than those who talk splendidly and raise clouds of dust to herald their approach. Of course, we need to put forth effort...

The last of Flynn's private letters to Nell to survive was written early in 1919 and was labelled "Personal" and "sub rosa". He was in a fix—mixed signals had resulted in Minnie Kinnear being appointed to Beltana although Flynn had earlier promised the posting to Nell. Flynn was prepared to ask Minnie to move again after six months to fulfil his commitment to Nell. He said he would do so if Nell was determined to serve at Beltana, but might she consider going to Port Hedland instead? It might even prove more beneficial to go far from home, as it had in the case of Abraham, who was ordered out of his parents' land: "Therein lay the method of his growth in character and power".

Then Flynn turned to answer questions of Nell's regarding tragedies in the lives of young friends of hers. Nell had been rocked by losing two close friends. One friend she had nursed until death; the other, "Prince", had died from the influenza that ravaged the world after the war. Once again, Flynn attempted to impart his own approach to tragedy to his young protégée. He took an eternal viewpoint:

> Your friend's case was indeed sad, and inscrutable to us. But we have to look right into the blackest sin, and the most exquisite <u>innocent</u> suffering alike, and go on with a smile and a cheer and a song. Anyhow, "<u>That</u> (heaven) is the reality, <u>this</u> is the Dream", wipes out most suffering from an <u>ultimate</u> view".

It is interesting how regularly Flynn's advice to Nell progressed to a spiritual plane. Nell subsequently found it hard to comprehend when hearing criticisms of him as "not spiritual enough". She felt sorry for Flynn when a friend told her he had seen Flynn struggling to put on a "dog collar" outside an Assembly meeting, saying: "Perhaps they will think I am a bit more spiritual". Those who knew him well discovered his prayer life and inner life were deep and, as Fred McKay said: "Flynn was a one-off and so was easily misunderstood because he did not fit the mould. But I found the Holy Spirit to be with him in a unique way. And I heard him once, late at night, praying for the AIM, mentioning each one who served in turn by name."

Later, in 1919 in the *Australian Inland Mission Weekly Notes*, Flynn announced that Nell, with her sister Nancy working as her "companion", would relieve Sister Simpson at Port Hedland in the spring. At last his protégé was ready to serve! He wrote further a jocular appreciation of Nell and the Triple Alliance:

> Just about eight years ago, a letter reached the manse at Beltana, explaining that the writer was one of the senior girls at Port Adelaide and had joined with two others in a "Triple Alliance". The object of this new force was to do everything in their power for Oodnadatta Hospital. They did fine work too toward the fitting up—the hostel was then being constructed. Now the style of handwriting, and the "ginger" in sentiment expressed, led to further conference; in due course the secretary of the Triple Alliance announced her intention to train as a nurse. She was too young to start, but that was a defect that could be remedied in time...

Nell intended to take along her younger sister, Mary, as paid companion. She and Mary shared a natural affinity and similar sense of fun, such as the lifelike spider they would drop from the ceiling on a thread in front of new visitors to the family. Mary became engaged, though, so Nance opted to take her place. Nell was concerned at this, as Nance was the sloppiest of her sisters and nursing demanded good hygiene and a disciplined, responsible approach to duty. Nance was not consistent in these areas and could also be lazy at times. Nell anticipated a few familial problems.

Nell had a personal briefing session with Flynn that was to prove very influential. Basically, he told her to serve others as Christ would and to "placard Christian love" through her nursing, not allowing any discrimination against patients for conviction, colour or creed. Everyone was to receive the same love and care.

So it was that in September 1919 she set out with Nance by train and ship to face the challenges of Port Hedland. Friends had teased her with: "You're only going to Port Hedland to find a husband" and she had hotly denied this. Little did she know.

She found the cottage hospital there to be just that, a bungalow with a wide hallway to divide the Men's Ward from the Women's Ward and a series of smaller rooms to act as surgery and their bedrooms. It was so hot, though, around 40°C, that they and some patients slept out on the verandas to take advantage of the breezes blowing off the sea. Biting insects troubled them out there unless the breeze was up: "I am learning to rise early—often it's a case of being driven out of bed by mosquitoes and sandflies."

Sister Simpson handed over to Nell on 10th October and immediately Nell was flat out, mainly because the dreaded Dengue fever had struck the community. Where possible, Nell went out to nurse patients in their own homes, especially the children, but the more serious cases were taken into the hospital.

Then came the first of a series of tragedies. Mr Meiklejohn, the fatherly secretary to the nursing home, was caught by the tide, renowned for the speed at which it rushes in at Port Hedland. Flynn described the circumstances later on in the *Inlander* (1920):

> While out "dry shelling" near Port Hedland, Mr Meiklejohn mistook the time and the tide caught both him and a young companion. He ordered the latter to swim ahead as fast as he could, apparently with the deliberate intention of preventing a futile effort by the lad to save him, for he must have sunk immediately after. He left a widow and family who remain at Port Hedland.

That widow and family stayed with Nell and Nance in the hospital, trying to recover from their shock. Having lost her boyfriend and two close friends shortly before going to Port Hedland, Nell was able to comfort and counsel them effectively. Regarding tragedy, Flynn had told her its "chief value is so that we can help others" and she saw that clearly now.

That Sunday, Nell felt very sick. She asked the government doctor to come and tend some of the patients, as she was too ill. Fortunately, he had returned from Marble Bar where he spent Wednesday to Friday each week—sometimes longer—and so was able to help out a little at the hospital.

Her diary entries describe succinctly what followed:

> SUNDAY 2/11/1919: Dr came and minded patient while I slept. Feeling horrible; onset of Dengue! Dr insisted I should go to bed at night and give patient a bell.
> MONDAY 3/11/1919: Nance feeling funny, temp 103 or so. Dengue! Put her to bed. That's the chorus now [i.e. both of them had Dengue].
> TUESDAY 4/11/1919: Face like a balloon and scarlet
> WEDNESDAY 5/11/1919: Hands like beetroot
> THURSDAY 6/11/191: Hands and face still covered with rash
> FRIDAY 7/11/1919: Body covered with rash

Slowly, tortuously, she recovered—and so did Nance. What she did not mention, perhaps was too sick to write about, was that she had to continue to nurse the patients despite feeling ghastly herself—hers was a seven-day per week job and there was simply a limit to how much support the busy government doctor could give her. Furthermore, all her hair fell out during this period because of the Dengue fever. There was no withdrawing to hide her embarrassment as her duties were too frenetic and public, nor did she have a wig. Despite feeling and looking like death, she soldiered on with extraordinary grit and dedication.

Nell's hair did grow back slowly, but never fully, and remained thin thereafter.

After another episode of sickness, she went to a nearby station to recuperate for a few days. Unfortunately a horse kicked her and opened up a gash on her cheek. The river was flooding and she could not return to the doctor for help, so had to sit down in front of a mirror and stitch up her cheek unaided! Because of the way her image was reversed, this was very difficult and painful.

Nell had had a baptism of fire at Port Hedland.

Her diary shows that she continued to write to Flynn and receive replies, but this correspondence has not survived. However, we see her purposefully putting into practice the principles her mentor had already given her. For example, Flynn had said to her, "While you are out there, don't try to make Presbyterians of people. You will find that all denominations will come for help and they will go back to the city and their own churches. By your example, you must promote the cause of Christ, not denominationalism."

Nell followed this advice and went further, promoting the merging of denominations from then on. "Living in the bush you realise how superficial it is to go to different denominations. While we were in Port Hedland the new hospital was built and we had a 'popular girl' competition to see who could raise the most money. The girl who won it was a Roman Catholic. No one took any notice of this as it was just taken for granted. There was no division in the town itself; the Catholic children used to come to our Sunday School."

She records an interesting example where a denominational approach could have been disastrous. A poor but pleasant Catholic came for the amputation of his hand, ashamed that he could not afford treatment but desperate for help. Nell records that when the subject of his Catholicism came up the patient got the wrong end of the stick:

> The old chap thought I wanted to put him out because he was not of our denomination. I explained that we were there to help. And the doctor was very good when the amputation was done, took hand measurements, etc., got all the gadgets he needed and sent them to me to give to the man.
>
> The patient then told me that he wanted to leave the hospital, but he wasn't well enough because it is a big shock having an amputation. I said: "Mr Olsen, you stay here, it is not very satisfactory to us after we have had a successful operation if you go, so you stay here"—and he did until he had recuperated sufficiently.

Flynn had also asked her to be aware that the AIM would be judged by her actions and standards. Nell took this so literally that she would not even dance when attending local parties and balls. Flynn had not meant her to follow such a stringent lifestyle and many of the young nurses at other of his cottage hospitals socialised in a more relaxed manner than did Nell, but this rigorous application of an instruction from Flynn was typical of her. It was only when she was about to leave in September 1922 and had become engaged to be married that she allowed herself to be seen dancing with her fiancé, Niel Campbell, who was the local stationmaster. She intended to return to marry him and live in Port Hedland in the April of the following year.

Did marriage mean Nell's contribution to Flynn's work would cease? Not at all. She would make herself available in Port Hedland to help out from time to time at the hospital. She also intended to become active in raising money for the mission. She was, and would always remain, an ardent supporter of Flynn's work.

Surprisingly, the focus of the Inglis sisters' contribution to Flynn's mission turns now to Nance.

Nance had not had an auspicious beginning to her service as paid companion to Nell. As anticipated, Nance would rather socialise than finish her chores. And when she did do them, as often as not they weren't done satisfactorily. So Nell had begun early on to exert some sisterly discipline and demand certain necessary standards. This was against Nell's gentle nature but she carried the overall responsibility for the hospital and could not do it all herself. After some tension and lots of discussion and prayer, Nance grudgingly began to toe the line. Over the years Nance would recognise this as a turning point in her life. Not only did Nell's nursing in Port Hedland inspire her to become a nurse, but the firm discipline Nell exercised gave her certain personal skills that were vital. She reminisced: "If it had not been for Nell's training and discipline in Port Hedland, I would never have lasted through my own nursing training later on."

So an inspired Nance began her training to become a nurse in 1923, aged 22. She also began a sporadic correspondence with Flynn, but on a more professional and less personal basis than Nell's. He reinforced her decision to start her training rather late in life compared to the others in her course:

> Between ourselves, it is a too common idea that "to make any good out of a woman you must catch her before she acquires any ideas of her own". Our theory is the very opposite. We are doing our best to persuade older women to enter training, and thus we hope to have a band of extra-strong workers later on.

She completed her general certificate in 1926 and then, on Flynn's advice, went to Narracoorte District Hospital as a charge nurse to obtain her Midwifery qualifications. He felt this would be a good preparation for serving at Alice Springs, for which he was grooming her. Doctor Keith Pavy commended her work there in these words: "She has discharged her duties efficiently and pleasantly, is very keen and thorough in her work and has been well liked by all the patients and staff and Medical Officers. Her character and habits are excellent and she has made many friends during her stay in Narracoorte." The lazy and sloppy girl had come a long way.

Nance found Alice Springs to be very different from Port Hedland. For a start, there were only twelve women in the town but lots of men, white and black. There was also no doctor and Nance had to make diagnoses and decisions about treatment that deeply concerned her. What if someone should die because she had made a misdiagnosis? She was only a nurse after all.

Then the railway line reached Alice Springs at last, amidst great fanfare and rejoicing. Nance wrote in October 1929 for the *Inlander* describing an incident associated with that first train:

> At 7 p.m. we started for Barron, arriving there at 2 a.m.— 120 miles. The man was fairly sick, so brought him down, arriving at Alice Springs at 9 p.m.—dosed him and waited. He did not improve.
>
> We knew a doctor from Adelaide was coming on holiday, so got in touch. He came on the first train, prepared to operate.
>
> Alas! We have no steriliser, no operating table, *no lots of things* when it comes to operations! We baked bundles all day, and had things in readiness, but it made us quake when we thought how doctor had everything ready for him in Adelaide. We raised the little hospital ward table for an operating table.
>
> A friend had kindly sent up a number of necessary little things, and the doctor's bag was full of surprise packets, much to our relief. He said the man was lucky—so far all is going well.
>
> Numbers of other people were waiting around hoping for advice. Doctor was very good to them all—refused to charge anyone; wasn't that kind of him? Among other patients two had teeth out, so we will not forget the first train to Alice Springs.

Flynn, as the editor, added a comment of his own: "The doctor travelled up with a friend, who was also a doctor, who helped him. The operation over, they presented their instruments to the Home, so that any future doctor happening by would find them at hand if needed. Such acts need no comment. The patient is now feeling quite fit."

The train was called "The Ghan" in honour of the "Afghan" cameleers, who had supplied Alice Springs so successfully for so many years. The Ghan brought many tourists to the Centre and the number of "blow-throughs" requiring treatment swelled. Nance's value as a frontier nurse grew rapidly as her experience widened.

Nance and Jessie Cavanagh fought an influenza epidemic that swept through the Centre in December 1929. Working day and night for weeks, they became totally exhausted. But their battle was successful and they did not lose any patients in the hospital. However, six Aboriginal prisoners in the local gaol died, perhaps through inadequate diet or lack of proper care, because no white prisoners died. Jessie and Nance had been called in to help towards the end and went in with food and basic medicines. Two sick but surviving prisoners had their sentences cancelled and disappeared—fate unknown.

These deaths in the prison upset Nance. She was in Alice Springs from 1928 to 1930, but was relatively happy to leave and take up a position at a hospital in Barmera. Neither she nor Flynn at that point could have imagined that she was destined to become the longest-serving nurse in the AIM network.

Nell and Niel, meanwhile, had moved to Esperance in 1925 when he was appointed Stationmaster there. Flynn visited them and was surprised to find his photograph on the mantelpiece, where Nell always displayed it. They ate juicy fruit from the ornate brass bowl that he had given them for a wedding present. He spoke for hours about his dreams for Flying Doctors and a wireless network and how the wealthy H.V. McKay was also enthusiastic.

Niel and Nell were inspired by Flynn's visit. They raised a great deal of money in support of his dreams and continued to do so throughout their lives.

But then a very personal tragedy struck the Campbells; Nell had a stillbirth from toxaemia in October 1926. This was a particular blow as they wanted a family and she was now 34 and Niel was 60. Nell became depressed by the loss and determined that something be done about the lack of medical facilities at Esperance. She contacted Flynn and asked him to do something.

John Flynn, moved by the personal tragedy of his friend, listened sympathetically to her plans for a hospital there. Although his resources were already overstretched, he agreed to provide paid AIM nurses providing the local community raised sufficient funds to build a hospital. The Government came to the party and set the figure to be raised as £1000, at which point they promised to provide a building.

Nell was determined. She approached others and they formed a local Women's Auxiliary to raise the necessary money. In Flynnian tradition, Nell went around the small community and garnered the support of any who were interested. The gregarious Mrs Daw, wife of a local shopkeeper, offered tremendous vocal support to the endeavour and gave it a high profile in the community. Slowly, the Auxiliary achieved the figure. The Government, stingy with the onset of the Depression, offered them the doctor's residence as their hospital. This was far too small and unsuitable in other ways, so Nell influenced the residents to refuse it. A stalemate resulted.

Meanwhile, the doctor in Esperance roped her in to nurse for him, telling her he would not have a "Sarah Gamp" while there was a registered nurse in town. (The term Sarah Gamp was applied to a woman who, without training as a midwife, went into private houses to assist with deliveries.) Never able to say "no", Nell soon found herself overworked. So when she fell pregnant again, Niel wisely insisted they escape to their little cottage at Kalamunda, near Perth, for four months so that she could rest up before and after the birth. He took long-service leave. Jean, their only surviving child, was delivered successfully and was a lusty, happy baby.

Nell's zeal to found an AIM hospital was undiminished by her own successful confinement.

Mr Ewan of the Health Department next offered the committee a hospital building that was about to be closed down. Nell was indignant and went to see him to tell him that they had been promised a new hospital and not a second-hand one. He suggested she see it first before rejecting it, as they would throw in all the furnishings, linen and equipment. That was a huge incentive. She contacted the committee and asked them to agree to nothing until she had seen it herself.

She subsequently travelled to the redundant hospital in the company of Mr Ewan. On inspecting it closely, she decided it would be fine for Esperance. The Government moved the building for them and it became the AIM Hospital at Esperance in January 1930.

Nell served briefly in the hospital in Esperance during 1931 when there was a staff shortage there, but then she answered a plea for help from her sister-in-law whose private hospital had been hit hard by the Depression. So Nell went to Frankston, Victoria, to run St Pancras Hospital. Niel finished up and followed shortly behind her, having just retired at 65.

John and Jean Flynn visited the Campbells and stayed at their home in Frankston. Jean Whimp, their daughter, was just four but remembers the adults spending many hours talking late into the night. She also remembers how Jean Flynn showed her how to dry her back after a bath, by herself, by using the towel diagonally.

Nance, meanwhile, served in the AIM Mitchell Home in Beltana from 1932 to 1934, with her friend and cousin Sister Elsie Sim as her "chum". Unexpectedly, while there, Nance was to play a part in helping one of Flynn's more expansive dreams to come true.

It began when she escorted five outback children to Adelaide to receive an award known as "The Banner" at the Assembly celebrations. Boisterous and fun-loving herself, she had vicarious enjoyment watching the great time these bush kids had during their week there. It suddenly struck her how valuable it would be to bring needy children from up North to the city for a holiday during which they could have medical checkups.

Flynn had been pondering the needs of children in the bush ever since his time at Beltana. He was appalled by the deprivations suffered by some children in the outback, socially and medically. One incident that upset him involved sick children who had been left to shelter inside a metal water tank, which must have become like a furnace during the heat of the day. And already, in his first letter to Nell, we see his sensitive concern that bush children not be made to feel inferior by their more sophisticated cousins in the cities. He said later: "We must help to bridge the gap between their brooding, isolated world and the modern city because many of them will go to the cities to live one day. They must also be socialised. Many have never played with other children besides brothers and sisters, if they are fortunate enough to have them." He shared his concerns with Patrol Padre Fred Patterson, who had been thinking along similar lines since 1931. Patterson proposed holding seaside camps for deprived children.

On Flynn's advice, Patterson contacted Nance and found she was enthusiastic. He asked her to prepare a report since she had some experience with taking bush children to the city.

We allow Flynn to take up the story from that point:

> Sister Inglis reports that here are thirteen children at Beltana in poor health, who would be very greatly benefited by a holiday at the seaside. Most of the fathers of these children, unfortunately, are out of work...This report from Sister Inglis indicates that the need for some health scheme such as the Far West Children's Scheme [of New South Wales], is essential. It also indicates how great are the difficulties. But, if the interest of the public is aroused, there should be little difficulty in financing holidays for children who are ill, but whose parents are non-financial.

Nance's report helped to launch, in 1933, the inaugural Inland Children's Camp, held at Glenelg near Adelaide. It was run and funded by the AIM and Fred Patterson led it and did most of the organising. It was a great success for the 35 children who attended and became an annual event. (Years later, after Flynn's death, a similar health scheme to the one suggested by Nance was launched by the AIM at their facility at Warrawee. This was called "The Far North Children's Health Scheme of the AIM" and did wonderful work for a number of years.)

With her sister-in-law's hospital back on its feet again, Nell and Niel returned to Esperance. Nell became Matron of the AIM Hospital in Esperance from 1935 to 1937. Niel, as a retired accountant, gave his services freely and also helped to collect bad debts as the hospital had been struggling financially. Nell got the Women's auxiliary functional again. She organised weekly needlework evenings by the light of kerosene lamps and linen items were made for hospital use and to sell to raise funds. Jean was now old enough to join in and enjoyed making things. She was also able to rejoice with her Mum when very sick people returned to health and to empathise with sad cases, like the little boy her age whose parents did not do anything about an infection caused by a fish hook until he was convulsing with tetanus and Nell could not save him. Jean perceived, further, that her Mum worked too hard and was often out late at night, resulting in exhaustion. It was no surprise, asked whether she would become a nurse one day, that Jean answered firmly in the negative.

Nell, with her church and nursing background, had a strong aversion to drunkenness, which she saw destroying many lives and family relationships. When Niel's supervisor came for dinner, he always seemed to imbibe more than Nell felt comfortable about. So later on in the evening she filled his beer bottle with cold tea! Either he was too polite or too inebriated to notice, but nothing was said. This became one of her favourite stories.

Yet her stance against alcohol never took precedence over her caring for people. For example, Niel's brother would come to stay but would sometimes return late at night "under the weather". Rather than face Niel's censure, he would implore Nell to let him in very quietly. Because of the plea in his voice, she always did, and did not tell Niel the following day. With Nell, love always triumphed over censure and characterised her whole approach to life.

Nell resigned as matron of Esperance hospital in 1938, aged 45, partly because of overwork. She continued to support the AIM and Flynn at every opportunity.

From the mid-1930s, Flynn had serious problems at Adelaide House, the AIM hospital in Alice Springs. Some involved blow-throughs who abused the services on offer and gave nothing in return. Most problems, however, stemmed from the rapid development of the region, making the mission hospital too small for the increasing volume of patients. Also, the local committee could no longer raise sufficient funds and folded.

Misunderstanding and recriminations resulted between Adelaide House and the community it wished to serve, although a few locals continued their support by spasmodically cutting wood for the stove or boiling sheets, towels and pyjamas in a copper. Otherwise the overworked Sisters cooked for the patients as well as doing the laundry and cleaning. Living in the same building, they had little privacy and were always on call and never off duty, *arranged Christmas celebrations...*

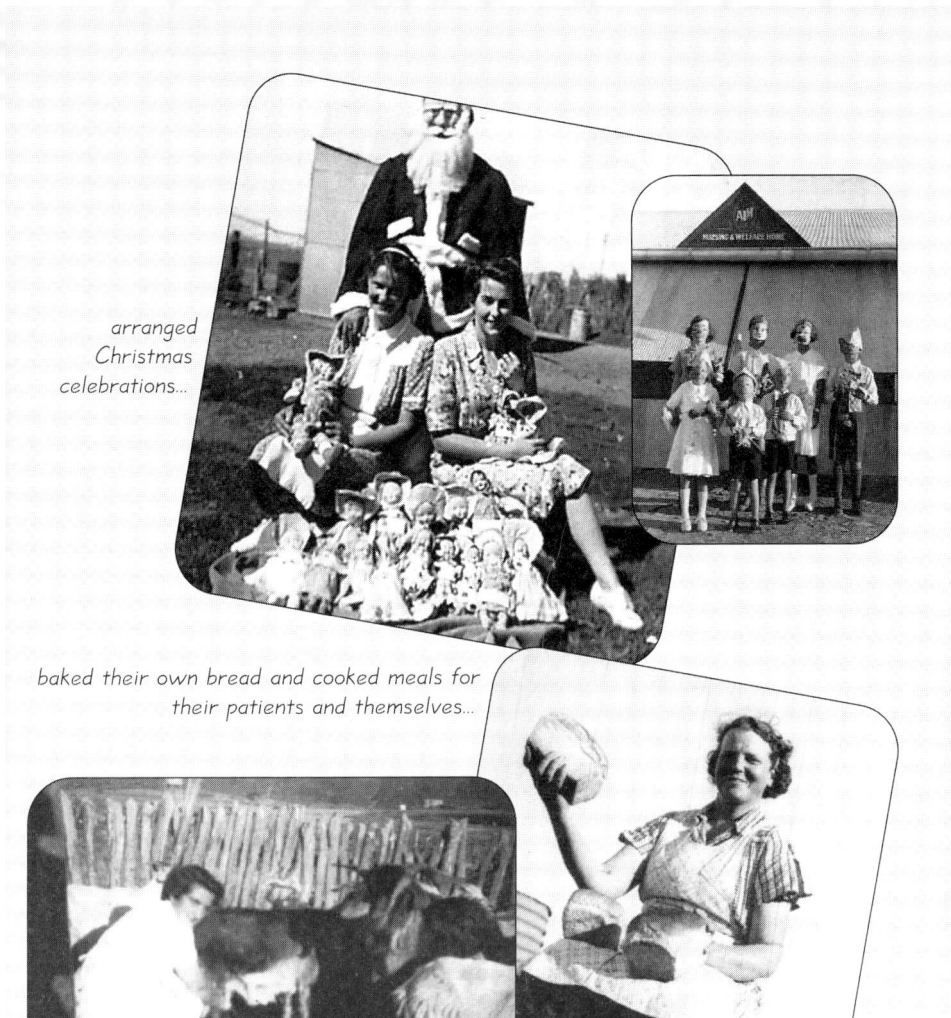

baked their own bread and cooked meals for their patients and themselves...

milked goats...

were on duty at the races...

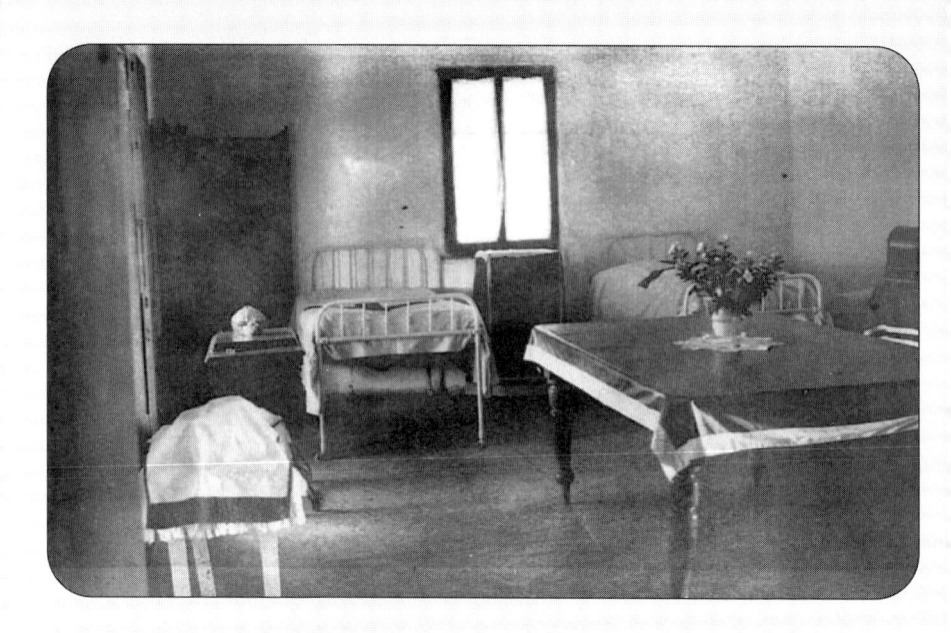

cleaned, polished, made beds and did the laundry, often with Aboriginal help, to keep their hospitals spic and span (Ward at Halls Creek, 1923)...

and always they improvised. Olive Bennett "gives the battery" to a stiff joint at Halls Creek in 1924. Note the wire-netting basket filled with scrap iron to provide traction to a limb. With a pen-knife and caustic fluid, Olive once carried out a successful operation by following a doctor's instructions relayed by telegraph.

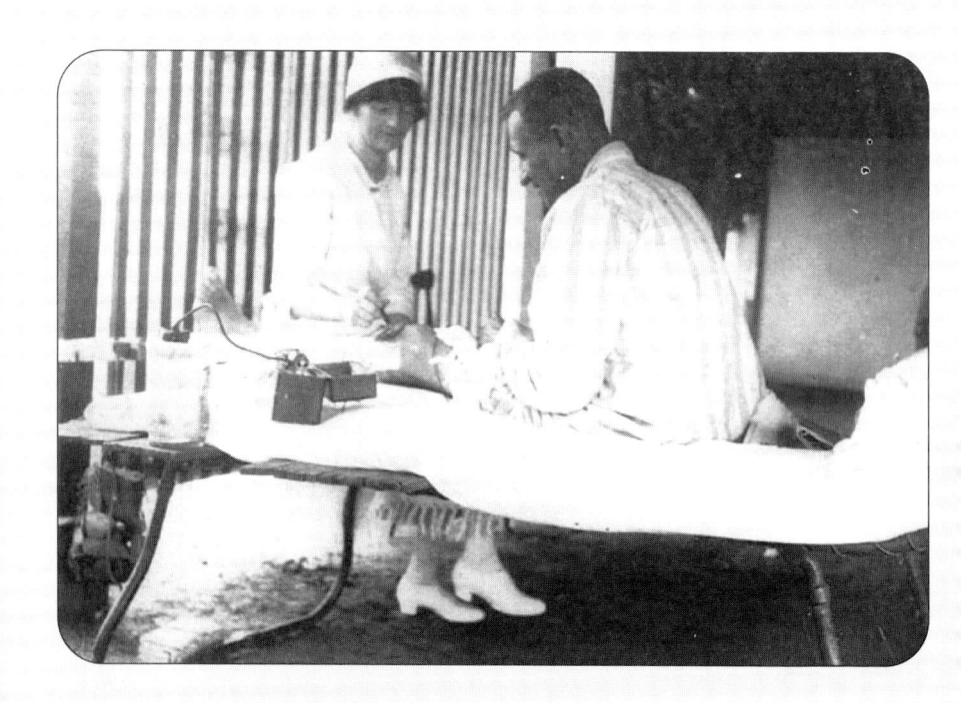

Nurses at Play

John Flynn was adamant that the nurses must socialise and become part of the community

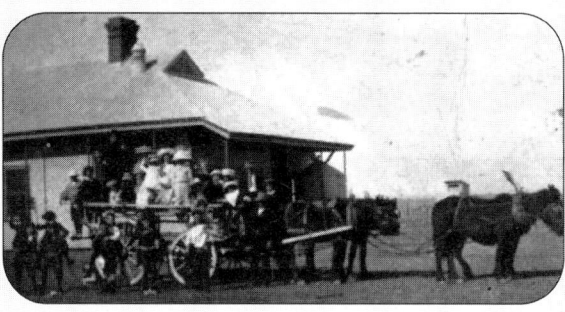

and they went on picnics (above), often with the whole town...

played sports...

went swimming (below), especially during long droughts, when water supplies at the hospital were too precious to allow bathing.

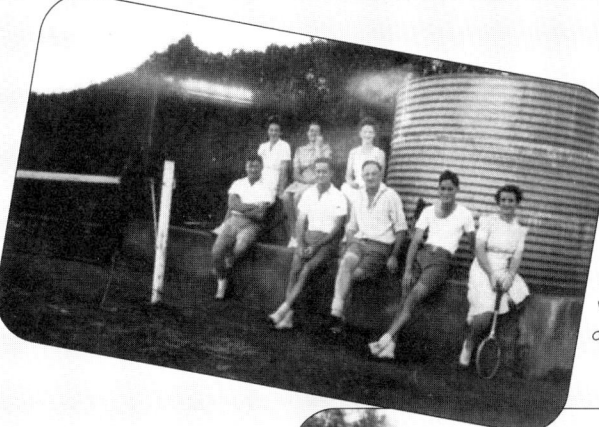

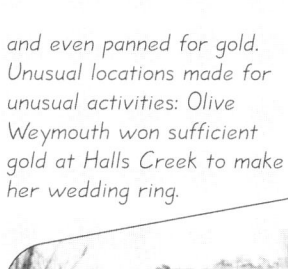

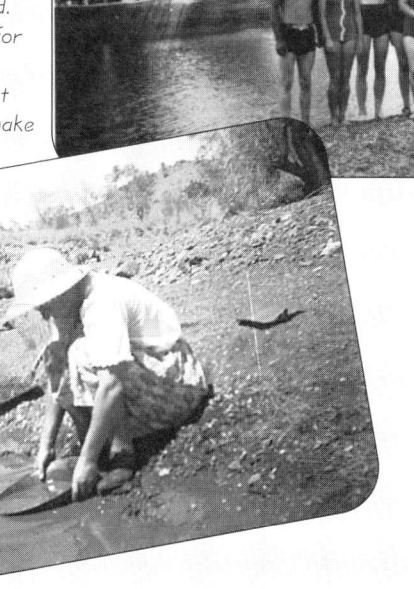

and even panned for gold. Unusual locations made for unusual activities: Olive Weymouth won sufficient gold at Halls Creek to make her wedding ring.

An Inland Miscellany

At Birdsville, time was often measured in terms of the Sisters' service: "Oh, that was during Sister So-and-so's time". When this photo was taken in 1936, the McLean-Bishop era was about to be replaced by the Cooper-Anderson era. From left: Edna McLean, Alice Anderson, Lillian Cooper and Amy Bishop.

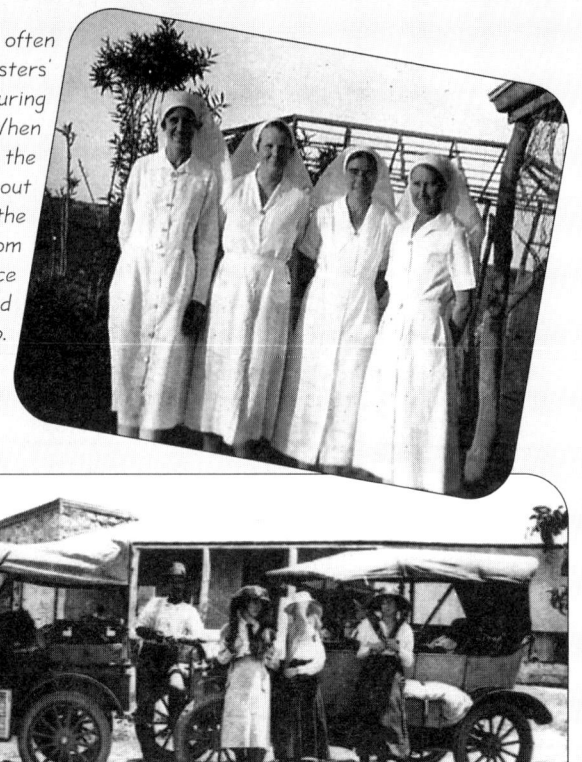

The annual picnic race meetings were extremely popular and people would travel many hundreds of kilometres to attend. The dances and opportunities for socialising more than compensated for the crude facilities. The photo above shows a group leaving for the Innamincka races in 1930 and pictured below is the Birdsville racetrack in 1936.

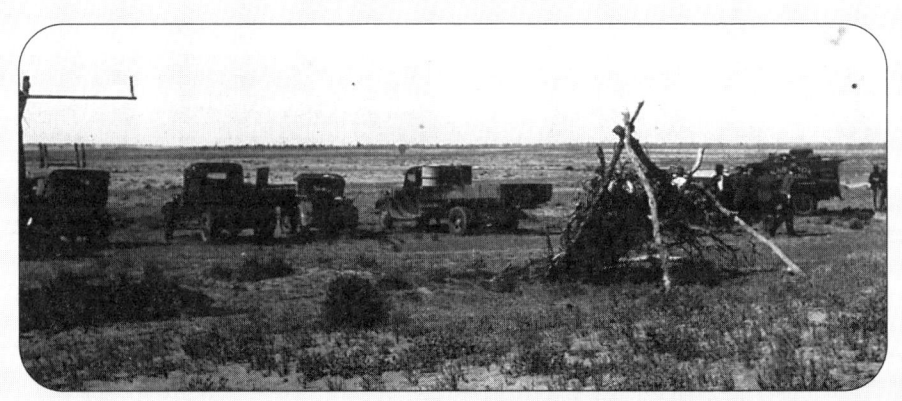

The Hospitals
"...like a bushman's pocket-knife"

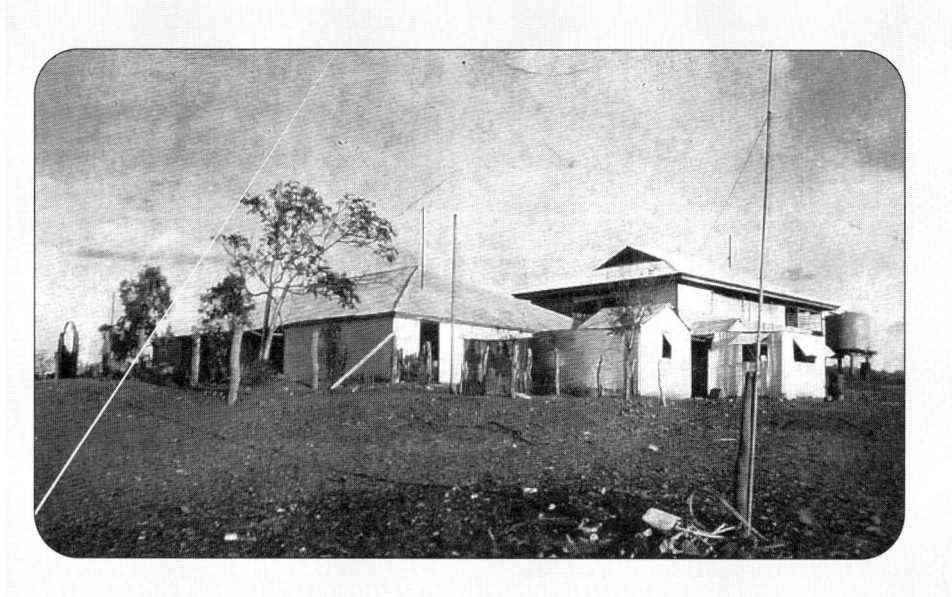

A front view of the Hospital at Halls Creek and, below, how it looked from the rear. In the foreground is the toilet; rudimentary but adequate.

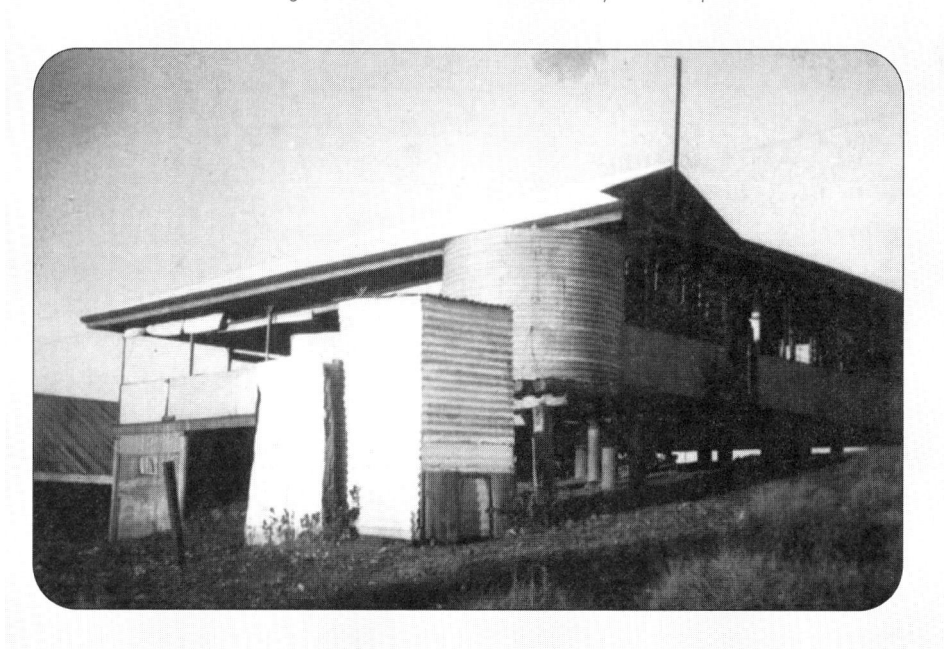

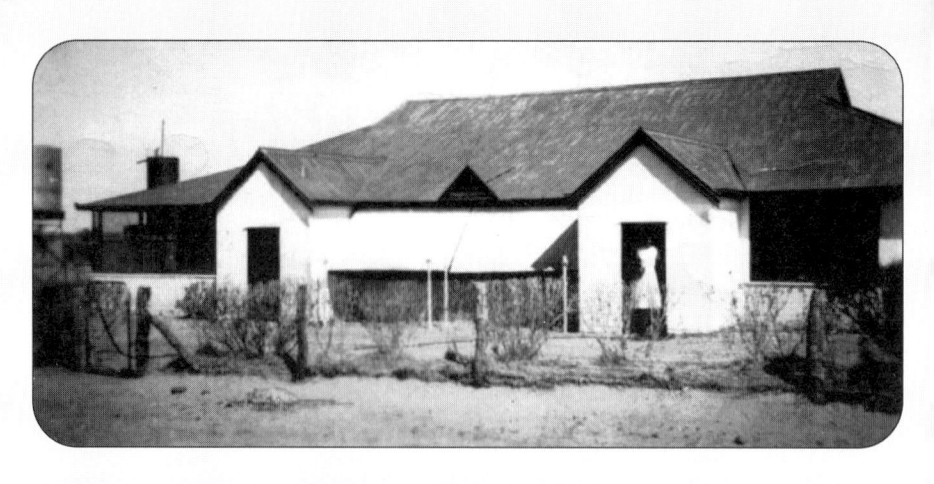

Above: The "new" Birdsville Hopital, overseen by Fred McKay and finished in 1937. Flynn said: "Instead of having an elaborate building ...we desired an institution like a bushman's pocket-knife that could be put to any use."

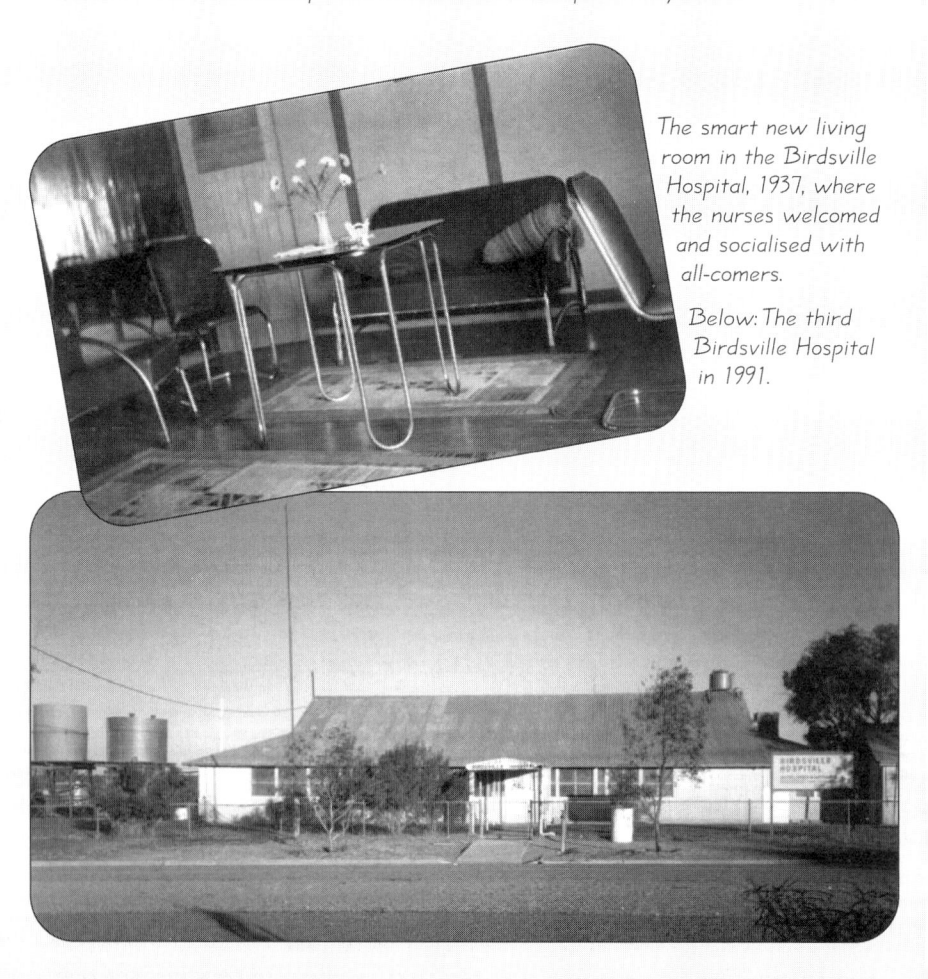

The smart new living room in the Birdsville Hospital, 1937, where the nurses welcomed and socialised with all-comers.

Below: The third Birdsville Hospital in 1991.

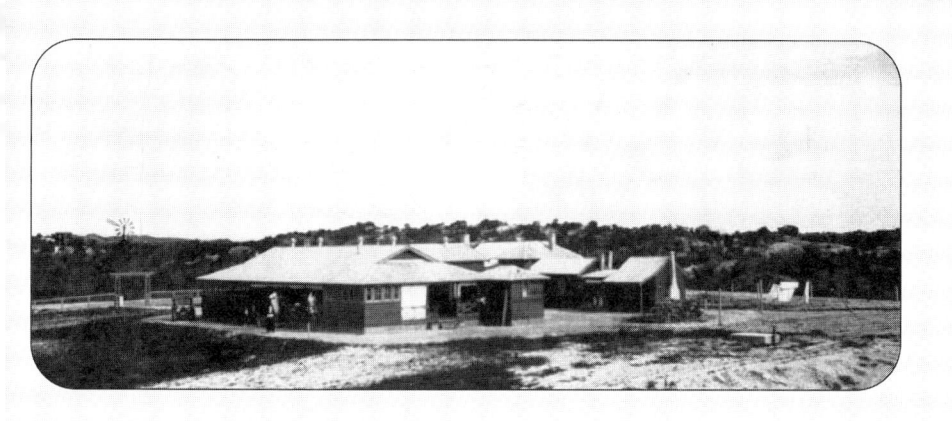

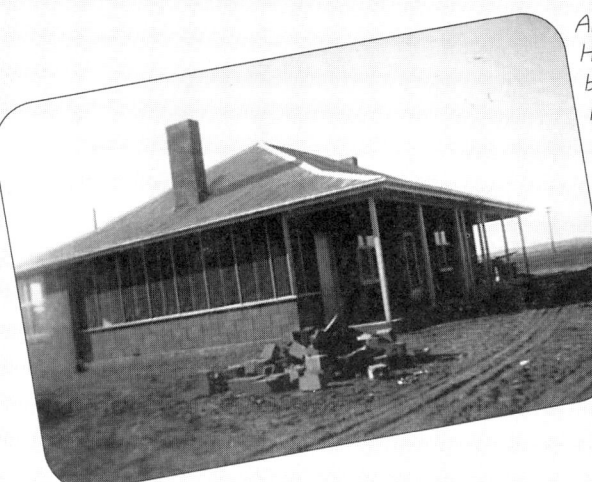

Above: The Esperance Hospital, WA, in 1930. Its building was inspired by Nell Inglis's determination. She garnered Flynn's support as well as that of the community, and served as its matron from 1935 to 1937.

Left: Over time, the buildings became simpler. Leigh Creek, SA, 1944.

Below: Lake Grace Hospital. The nurses' living quarters were upstairs.

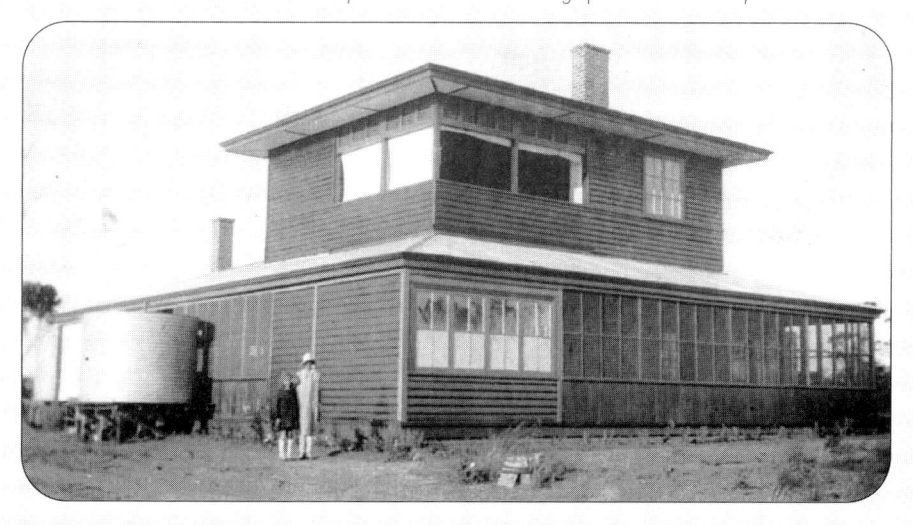

Trials of Inland Life

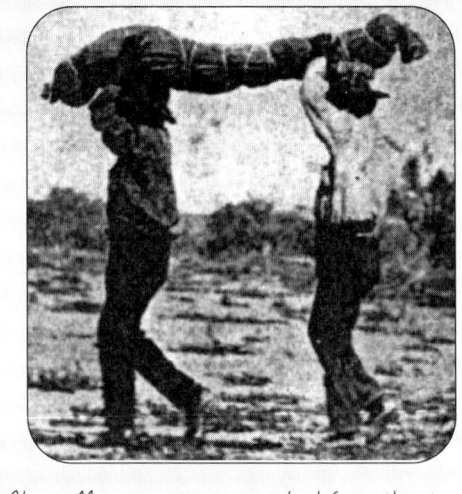

Above: Men sometimes perished from thirst and the Sisters would organise the burial service. If a coffin was unavailable, the body was shrouded in blankets or a swag.

Left: A duststorm could bring the desert to the door.

Below: The nurses were amazed at the improvisations used in emergencies. Here an injured man is ferried across the Diamantina in a boat made of canvas wrapped round packsaddles.

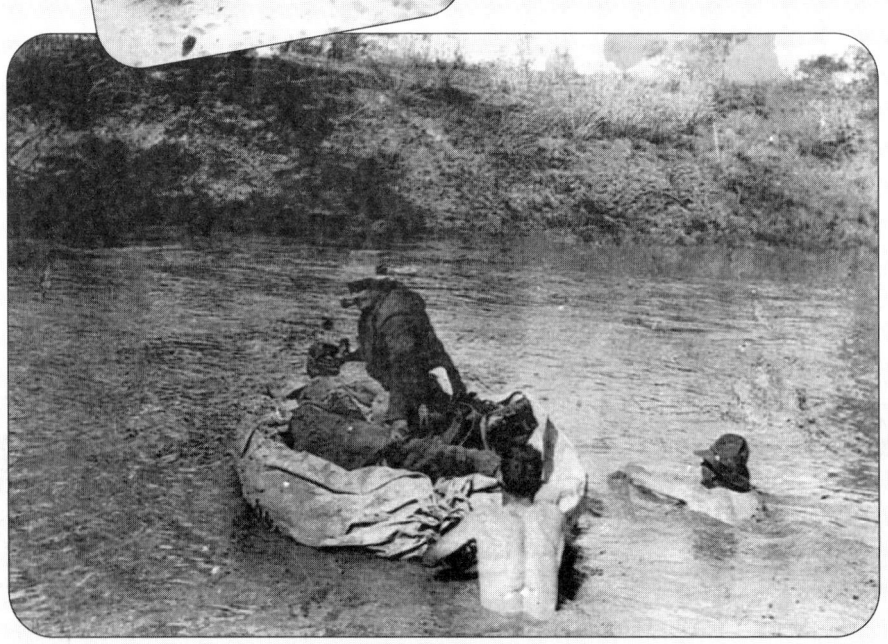

seven days a week. Patients came at any hour of the day or night as suited them; making prior appointments was not something done in the bush. Short on sleep and overworked, the Sisters became very stressed. Without sufficient funds, when there was an emergency call, a Sister would seek the support of local clergy to provide a vehicle to act as an ambulance while the remaining Sister carried all the load.

Flynn visited in 1934 to assess the situation. That same year the Sisters fought a diphtheria epidemic and a rampaging eye disease that left many locals, particularly Aborigines, visually impaired. Because it was highly infectious in nature, one nurse locked herself in with the infected patients until the epidemic abated. A third Sister came temporarily to lend a hand but the load remained overwhelming despite her being there.

A worried Flynn made representations to the Government to build a public hospital there with some urgency. If this approach of Flynn's sounds surprising, it was nevertheless in line with his vision of providing the best possible facilities for the bush. Flynn had always viewed his nursing homes as a temporary ministry to meet a desperate need, describing his approach in the 1927 *Inlander*:

> These institutions have met a crying need where widely-scattered pioneers have been unable to create the necessary organization. These "Homes" are really embryo public hospitals, i.e. they may be taken over by the residents when independent local management is made possible by further development... Meantime, they render much "social service" when nursing duties are not pressing.

The Minister of Health promised him that a modern government hospital would be built very soon, but they would need to hang on at Adelaide House until then.

Flynn needed someone special to rectify the degenerating state of affairs and regain full community support. He believed Nance alone could achieve this because she had been popular there and knew the local situation, so he asked her to go for his sake. He briefed her fully on the difficulties she would face. She accepted, fully realising it would be the greatest challenge of her life.

Nance went in 1937 with Sister Audrey Jaffer, and they had Sister Gibson to help in 1938 when the load once again became too much to bear.

Nance's strong character and organisational abilities soon had things on an even keel once more. Her buoyant, cheerful personality made her liked as well as respected. Greatly overweight by now, her whole body would shake when she chortled with mirth. And if a man became squeamish about an injection or some other treatment, she would threaten, "You keep quiet now and do as you are told, or I'll sit on you to hold you still." That threat always seemed to work.

Later Flynn wrote: "We can look back with pride, for the Sisters' letters show that however heavy the load and the human aggravation, they were remarkably uncomplaining. Sister Nance Inglis, who was serving a second term at Adelaide House those last two years, carried an incredible burden with cheerful dedication." High praise indeed from the great man! He also told Fred McKay years later how grateful he had been to "our famous Nan", whose friendship and skills he had relied on at Alice Springs. She had, indeed, achieved a remarkable turn-around for him.

Adelaide House had been the first and only hospital in all of Central Australia between 1926 and 1939. When it opened, there were around forty whites in the town as well as the Aborigines and it catered comfortably. By 1939 the town's population had leapt to over 1000 whites plus the Aborigines and the hospital was bursting at the seams, so it was no wonder that the Sisters were counting down the days until the government hospital would open on 14th February 1939.

Then there were delays—the furniture did not arrive in time and the rain cut the railway line, so the opening was put back to 20th May. However, the government nurse arrived in March and had nothing much to do, so Nance arranged the early transfer of their patients to the new hospital. Flynn in Sydney received this relieved telegram on 21st March:

> SISTER INGLIS TO INLANDER (AIM SYDNEY)
> ALL PATIENTS TRANSFERRED TO HOSPITAL TODAY

Sister Jaffer transferred over as well, but not Nance. Flynn had an exciting new concept for her to pioneer, about which she was most enthusiastic. That story belongs in Volume II, as do the later contributions these two fine sisters made to Flynn's work.

Many other AIM Sisters besides Nell Inglis formed romantic attachments while serving in Flynn's hospitals. The next chapter looks at some of their stories.

9

DIARIES AND ROMANCE AT ALICE SPRINGS

Flynn often had great difficulty finding suitable nurses to serve at his outposts. How might you expect he would react when they fell in love and married local men?

When I asked Fred McKay that question, he surprised me with his answer: "Oh, Flynn was delighted, providing they finished their term of service, which most of them did."

"I would have expected him to be annoyed."

"You have to keep in mind Flynn's vision, to brighten up the bush by encouraging family life. What better way than to have AIM nurses, wonderful girls, marrying and settling out there? They made first class wives. I remember counting them once and already more than thirty nurses had married men of the Inland. And you have to remember that most stayed out there and provided back-up nursing when we needed it."

"And the marriages were successful, in the main?"

"It appeared so. Oh, well, some of the matches were inappropriate, an educated nurse from the city marrying a nearly illiterate drover for example, especially if they tried to live in a city afterwards. Flynn told me some of these relationships developed in the outback because, he thought, sexuality increased at times in really hot tropical conditions and common sense didn't, but he added this was only a theory. At any rate, nearly all of the marriages appeared to be good."

"And what of Flynn himself? Was he ever interested in Sister Small, as a relative of hers has suggested to me?"

"I had not heard that." Fred's eyes narrowed slightly as he pondered this possibility. After a short delay, he continued, "Of course, he spent a long time with Sisters Nell Small and Ina Pope compared with other nurses, because he was building the hospital at Alice Springs and they were patching him up all the time, especially his hands, which would bleed through the bandages.

But he would carry on working regardless, so they had to chide him, something they found difficult because he was their boss. He ignored their good advice in order to get the hospital finished in time and his hands became badly infected. I remember him telling me years later, as a joke, that he had the honour of being the first patient in his own hospital. If he took a romantic interest in Sister Small it would not have gone far, I'm sure of that."

I was not so sure, so turned to the copy of Sister Small's diary that I have, to look for clues. Its faint script is hard to decipher. She met up with Flynn when he left the building project at Alice Springs to collect her and Sister Pope from Oodnadatta. It was 1926. There followed a difficult journey during which they were bogged a number of times and had other car trouble. Flynn was mentioned often but in the most prosaic terms:

> SUNDAY 16TH MAY: Helped Mr Flynn to get car out of hole. Delighted him when we moved a few inches. By 12 midday we got out. Mr Flynn took several snaps of car in bog. It was glorious to be in motion once more.
> TUESDAY 18TH MAY: Mr Flynn not at all well and right hand very swollen. Bashed it several times during day.

Similarly, once they arrived and settled in the new hospital, as yet unfinished:

> FRIDAY 21ST MAY: Went to the telegraph office with Mr Flynn.
> FRIDAY 28TH MAY: Evening at Mr Flynn's camp to listen to wireless, but not a success.
> SUNDAY 30TH MAY: Went for a short run (in his Dodge car) with Mr Flynn and party, after Sunday School.
> MONDAY 31ST MAY: When we got home around 10 p.m. Mr Flynn was waiting as per usual.

Soon afterwards another man is mentioned in her diary. It is the local policeman, Mr Littlejohn, who took her for a spin in his car after a "dance in the moonlight on the lawn which ended at midnight".

The diary ends, unfortunately, on Monday 28th June, so what happened next may never be told. But the penultimate entry mentions Flynn and tells a story all of its own:

> Mr Flynn drove us home and to our surprise called for us again. Had wonderful service, and communion after service, which was very impressive. We are wicked girls. Mr Flynn wanted to take us home and we did not know how to shake him off, as Mr Littlejohn wanted to take us out for a spin again with Phil Windle. It was very amusing to see Mr Littlejohn have a word with our "John", who bade us goodnight. I would like to know what happened. Went for a spin which freshened us up wonderfully.

Whether Flynn had been keen on Sister Ellen "Nell" Small is not apparent from these diary entries, but her feelings about him are. What we do know is that she later married Littlejohn and Flynn married his secretary, Jean Baird. Both marriages were very successful.

The second Sister at Alice Springs, Isabella "Ina" Pope, also married a local man, Billy McCoy. The McCoys did sterling work later among mixed-race children in Alice Springs. Both Ina and Nell continued to be enthusiastic supporters of Flynn's work and nursed in AIM homes from time to time.

Many of Flynn's nurses married while serving the AIM in some far-flung outpost and the locals joked that AIM stood for All In for Marriage. Romance can be bitter as well as sweet and others had their hearts broken. We find glimpses of both scenarios in the short extracts we take from Gwen McCubben's diary.

Gwen served in Alice Springs for two years, starting June 1930. Her colleague was Sister Florentine "Flo" Farmer.

Surviving accounts laud Gwen as an outstanding nurse with a good sense of humour. Her diary reveals the person behind the icon, that she was a normal woman who had squabbles and made mistakes. But her story illustrates an important truth in that Flynn's angels were angels because of their extraordinary dedication that triumphed over personal issues.

Among the first women at Alice Springs to befriend Gwen were Mrs Nell Littlejohn (nee Small) and Mrs Ina McCoy (nee Pope) and so the possibility of a similar romance must have been very obvious to her. However, demands on the nurses' time had become increasingly hectic and she was immediately very busy with little time to socialise. For example, her first real emergency happened just a week after arrival and proved to be stressful at the same time—the Stationmaster, Mr McDonald, had acute appendicitis and needed an operation. The only local doctor who could operate was on a camel tour among the hills. An alternative was to fly the patient to Port Augusta and there was a suitable aeroplane, but the two women passengers who were approached absolutely refused to give up their seats and wait for the next aeroplane, even if it meant the death of the patient. They explained haughtily that they had no clothes or shoes they could wear suitable for Alice Springs. Exasperated and disgusted, the policeman Littlejohn set off that night to look for the doctor in the hills. Gwen persisted in trying to arrange an evacuation by air as Littlejohn was unlikely to find the doctor in the dark, and eventually two men volunteered to stay behind. The plane flew out at 8 a.m. the next morning and the doctor and Littlejohn arrived a few hours later, but the medico graciously told her she had done the right thing and appeared not to be upset at having his holiday interrupted unnecessarily.

McDonald was operated on and his life saved.

To give some idea of Gwen's busy schedule, while Sister Farmer was away with Mr McDonald, I quote her record of in-patients for July 3rd, 1930:

> Miss Spinston, who has a sore throat, is up today.
> Mr Curtis, who has had some pleurisy, is improving.
> Mrs Scott is also much better and out on the veranda today.
> Mr Cuilidad, who has an infection of the middle ear, appears to be improving slowly.
> Bill Sullivan's lacerated hand is getting on well.
> His sister, Florence, has Argyrol in her eyes, which are now practically cured.

With many outpatients to nurse in addition, many of whom often "took anaesthetic at the Stuart Arms Hotel" before coming to have infected wounds treated or teeth removed, Gwen had little time to socialise. Her diary expresses tiredness and stress, without a hint of interest in the opposite sex.

However, things quietened down for a short period and both nurses took advantage of the many friendly invitations that were extended to them.

Gwen mentions Phil Windle for the first time on July 18th 1930, the same Phil Windle we met first in Sister Small's diary. It is an innocuous entry: "Intended writing letters but Mr Windle called. Had supper about 9.30 p.m." Phil was a young bachelor struggling to make a living. He operated a nearby repair "garage" and would fix cars and tackle almost anything mechanical—even aeroplanes were wheeled into his shed for repair from time to time.

Then another impossibly busy period followed, during which sickly twins were delivered who needed constant nursing.

> Only got 2 hours sleep last night and not any more tonight... Was up three times during the night with the babies... Our largest twin is very ill. In fact, we feel sure she is going to die... Baby no. 2 looked ghastly. Colour grey. Was up all night with her.

These twins had to remain in the hospital for months and, with the needs of two demanding babies added to their other duties, the nurses suffered from severe sleep deprivation. They were stressed and irritable. After a series of nights with just four hours of sleep, Gwen bemoaned: "I have Monday-itis and am afraid I am getting a bit morose. I am feeling quite easily upset today." Then a few days later, "We are not having many visitors now because we are too busy to entertain."

Both twins survived and were ultimately discharged, but only the following year, by which time the Sisters were very fond of them and found the parting difficult.

But from September, and as time allowed, Phil Windle became a regular visitor. Gwen's diary entries about him gradually changed in character:

> 7th SEPT: Farmer and I went for a walk with Mr Windle to Heavy Tree [sic] Gap.
> 10th SEPT: I went for a drive with Phillip about 20 miles south. [Note that she misspelled his Christian name at first, and sometimes both names.]

> 11th SEPT: Phillip came to supper again. We were practically without light until nearly 8 p.m.
> 29th SEPT: I am cook again and Flo nurse. Anyhow, it gives me a chance to see more of Phillip.
> 2nd NOV: Philip calls over every night. If he did not, I don't know what I would do, I am so used to seeing him now.
> 14th NOV: A favourite of Philip's:
>> Ah Love: could thou and I with fate conspire
>> To grasp this sorry scheme of things entire
>> Would not we shatter it to bits—and then
>> Remould it nearer to the heart's desire?

In some senses, this quote from *The Rubáiyát of Omar Khayyám* (translated by Edward Fitzgerald) was prophetic. Their romance faced a series of problems that threatened to shatter it.

Meanwhile, Flo had become interested in Tony Morgan. Gwen hinted as much as early as October, and when Tony came in for treatment on 2nd March 1931, with a gunshot wound to the eye, Gwen commented: "Now that Flo is nurse, he will get looked after very well."

When Tony had an operation to remove bullet fragments, Flo assisted and Gwen gave the anaesthetic. But Tony still required a lengthy recuperation in the hospital, allowing time for a romantic relationship with Flo to develop.

Romance makes people exclusive, and Gwen noted on 14th March: "It was the opening night of the new hall. Flo went for a few minutes. Philip and I did not go and I think the residents are rather disgusted with the three of us."

Tony was not in any hurry to leave the hospital, and we find him assisting Flo. On 18th March, Gwen wrote: "Peter sustained a compound fracture of the leg which Flo and Tony treated and stitched up."

While Tony and Flo's romance began to flower, Gwen and Philip entered a less certain stage. Excerpts from the diary enable us to follow the overall progress of both relationships:

> 19th MARCH: Philip came after tea and was feeling rather blue.
> 20th MARCH: I was not in a very good mood tonight. Felt rather depressed.

26th MARCH: Tony discharged. Flo has fallen pretty heavily for him. I hope it ends well and she does not get disappointed.

28th MARCH: Flo was out late with Tony and seems very happy.

29th MARCH: Philip called this morning but had very little to say. I spent a most miserable morning upstairs and was very sorry for myself. Philip and I went for a drive to Simpson's Gap and took our tea. We had quite a nice evening and afternoon. Flo and Tony went for a walk when we returned. I went to bed after they went. I don't know what time Flo returned.

30th MARCH: I feel rather blue, though in spite of all I know I think far more of Philip than I should, but I really cannot help it. Some drunken men were making a frightful noise at the hotel and Philip called to see whether the noise was coming from here, but did not come inside. I went to bed and left Flo and Tony up.

31st MARCH: Philip and I had morning tea together, as did Flo and Tony. The latter left for the bush per camel this a.m. Philip had a bet with me that Tony would not go, the bet being a bottle of cool drink. He brought the same and some chocolates with him at night. I feel a little less blue today but still there is a lot to think about.

7th APRIL: Tony returned. That finishes Flo. They spent most of the afternoon together. Philip came over.

9th APRIL: Flo and Tony spent most of the day in the sitting room.

10th APRIL: Another night alone and I feel very lonely. Philip never called and after setting the tray for Tony and Flo, I went to bed.

12th APRIL: Tony came as usual but stayed for dinner. Philip came to tea. We had a serious few minutes' talk before church. He seems so worried and I would like to help, but do not seem to be able to do much.

At this time, when Gwen and Philip's relationship was faltering a little, tensions arose between Tony and Philip, which spilled over slightly to Gwen and Flo.

5th MAY: Philip came at night and brought 2 tins of strawberries and cream, one for Flo and Tony which she refused because she said Philip did not like Tony and they would not have anything he bought. Philip and I had one tin between us. I got supper ready and Tony cleared off without having any and of course Flo had none either. I will be glad when he goes away. Flo seems quite different since he has been coming here. Of course he is not popular with anyone and she knows it.

6th MAY: Philip and I had the second tin of strawberries for supper. Flo got their own.

9th MAY: Tony came for morning tea. Philip never comes to tea now and never has supper. He called. Walked to the telegraph and Philip drove me home.

5th JUNE: Flo and Tony had tea together. Philip came over for the evening and we had a serious talk. I really don't know how things will end; the future sometimes looks like a great black cloud. This time next year we will know.

16th JUNE: Train left at 8.30 a.m. with Tony on board. Flo is missing him very much.

20th JUNE: I went to the telegraph with Philip to get the mail. Got about 8 letters. Flo got one from Tony. She also paid a visit to the telegraph this morning.

22nd JUNE: Flo got telegram from Tony.

26th JUNE (FRIDAY): Philip took the afternoon off because he thought it was Saturday and shot a few ducks. Came here at night and made me feel quite miserable for a time. Anyhow, I cannot help loving him and he is dearer to me than anyone else even with his faults.

4th JULY: Had another dance for the Hostel. Flo went but is terribly worried about Tony. He had an op last Thursday and is to have another on Monday. I got two wonderful nighties from Rene. They are much too nice to ever wear.

6th JULY: Flo is terribly miserable. She has been to the store three times to see if there is a wire for her. Had a serious talk with Philip last night. I wonder will things ever straighten out? But one is so helpless to do anything. I hope fate will be kind. He is so worried and perhaps I only increase his worries.

> 9th July: Flo is very miserable, waiting to hear how Tony is.
> 20th July: Saw Philip before breakfast, during the morning, after dinner and again tonight. He seemed a little despondent and cannot tell me yet what is causing it. The dear old thing! I just love every bit of him and would do anything at all for him. He talks of selling out and leaving the place, but I hope he does not until we leave too.

The nurses did not allow their personal lives to interfere with their duties and fought a number of interesting medical battles. Some were lost ("Doreen McDonald died about 9 p.m. Had been suspected of eating oleander leaves") and a great number more were won ("The twins, Margaret and Valmai, are 12 months today!"). Their other duties continued also, such as maintaining the gardens. *The Messenger* quoted an amusing situation in this regard:

> The Sisters at Alice Springs are proud of their vegetable garden. The crows have been after the eggs. Sister McCubben has not killed any, but has helped chase them into a corner, where someone else hit them on the head with a stick.

True to her compassionate nature, it was not Gwen doing the final despatching.

A new activity became the rage in town—listening to the wireless. One of the first sets was in the Hostel and despite variable reception would draw a crowd around it to enjoy programs broadcast from Sydney or Melbourne. And the glamour of wireless even became a courting bauble, as Gwen records with tongue in cheek:

> Had a visit from a man who promised to bring his portable wireless set tomorrow, also some tarts, and has promised me a ride in a plane on Sunday—and thinks he may marry me eventually.

Meanwhile, Flo and Tony's relationship seems to have faded and was not mentioned again in the diary. Flo remained unhappy for some time.

Gwen and Philip spent more time together now that Tony had left. Their relationship had typical ups and downs and neither seemed sure where it would end, although others in the town were not in much doubt: "Mrs Jones informed me that two men had told her I was engaged. It is wonderful how much people know about us."

Then an event occurred that was to prove pivotal—Philip went to Adelaide for some weeks to visit his family. Separations can make or break a romance, as had happened with Tony and Flo.

> 6th OCT: Philip has gone. He called to say goodbye and now I feel as though I have lost part of myself. I miss him dreadfully already, but still I should not be selfish – he must see his people sometime.
>
> 7th OCT: John Donnellan called and said Philip had asked him to keep an eye on me. I am sure there is no need because I love Philip too much to bother with anyone else.
>
> 9th OCT: I am still missing Philip very much. I think of him all day and dream of him at night.
>
> 10th OCT: In another week he will be home, I hope.
>
> 11th OCT: Yesterday I extracted two teeth from a man who had been drinking fairly well. He was so pleased with the operation that he broadcast it at the hotel. Within an hour he brought another patient down to have two teeth extracted. The second patient was quite drunk. I looked in his mouth—he had not a tooth in his head.
>
> 17th OCT: Philip did not return and I feel so miserable.
>
> 18th OCT: Had a letter from Philip. Feel much more cheered. Still, two more weeks is a long time!
>
> 19th OCT: Wrote five pages to Philip.
>
> 23rd OCT: Margaret has told Mr Partridge ["Skipper", one of Flynn's Patrol Padres] that Philip is not returning on this train. I don't know what I will do! Before Mr Partridge went home he decided I was taking it rather badly so told me the truth, that Philip is returning *by car*. It made a great difference. They all enjoyed themselves immensely teasing me. Anyhow, I don't care if the whole town knows I love Philip.
>
> 27th OCT: Philip may not return until next week. I wish I could hear something really definite, this suspense is just awful—no one knows what it is like!

> 28th Oct: Had a rather miserable day. Missed Philip very much.
>
> 30th Oct: Still no Philip. I never wished for anything more than I do for his return. I wonder, will he be on the train tomorrow?
>
> 31st Oct: The train came in about 10.15 p.m. and no Philip.
>
> 1st Nov: Mail arrived and most important of all—a letter from Philip, which cheered me very much. He will be home on Thursday 5th November, never to leave me again!
>
> 5th Nov: Dreamt about Philip all night. Thought he was home. He should come home today but I fear it may not be until tomorrow.
>
> 6th Nov: After dinner I was lying down and nearly asleep when I heard someone on the back veranda, and in a few moments Philip's head came around the door. I really do not know who was the most excited. It is just wonderful to have him back!

Philip's return heralded a new level of commitment between them.

Gwen's diary stops its daily record on 18th November. The next entry is 29th December, "Philip's birthday. I left for Adelaide". Then there was another hiatus until 5th March 1932. "I got my ring". It begins again towards the end of March and continues, daily, until early in May. Then there is another silence, until this final entry:

> Two new Sisters arrived to relieve us in August. *I married my Philip on August 15th.* John Donnellan and Sister Farmer were witnesses. Rev. Kingsley Partridge tied the knot.

Gwen and Philip lived in Alice Springs for many years. Phil prospered in his business. They lived on the property next to the Hostel, providing friendship and a helping hand to each of Flynn's nurses who came there to serve. They raised money for the AIM too and Phil served on the Hostel Committee. They were good members of the local church and Gwen sang at services and helped with Sunday School. And when Fred McKay needed their property for the John Flynn Memorial Church, they sold it to the

AIM "for a good price" and moved on. Theirs was an especially happy union.

* * * *

One problem Gwen and Philip had had was communicating over long distances when separated. With the advent of Flynn's pedal radio network, this problem was diminished to a degree, providing you were not shy that dozens of others might be party to your conversations. Alice Anderson and Lillian Stevenson were AIM nurses at Birdsville (1936–38) who used the airwaves for some "serious wooing".

"If you wanted to talk with your loved one, you had to pick your moment as everyone could listen in," remembers Lillian.

So Lillian and Alice hatched a cunning plan to obtain some privacy. They decided Morse code, which they had learned, could come in handy because most of the Inlanders were not fluent in it. They even managed to have some amorous conversations using it before they learned it had been cracked. Apparently a "listening party" at Marree would gather daily around their set, drinks in hand, to decipher the messages for a laugh.

Despite these setbacks, both these nurses ended up marrying the men who had courted them over the radio.

10

Territorian Heroes—Ruth Heathcock and Elsie Jones

Some of Sister Ruth Heathcock's life has assumed almost legendary status in the Northern Territory. The problem with legends is separating fact from fiction. Many pages have been written about her by a number of different authors, but unfortunately much of it is contradictory. I have not found an account either written or authorised by Sister Ruth herself, so I am relying as my benchmark on a short biography written by Reverend Arch Grant and a telephone conversation I have had with him. Arch, a man of the highest integrity, interviewed Sister Ruth herself in 1989 and, as one of Flynn's Patrol Padres, knew the areas involved. His biography appears in the *Northern Territory Dictionary of Biography, Volume 2*.

Another difficulty lies in the nature of Sister Ruth herself. She was a mystic and not given to attempting to explain everything.

Here, though, is some information about her intriguing life.

Ruth was born in South Australia in 1901. She spent her childhood near the shores of Lake Alexandria, making friends with the Aborigines of Point McLeay Mission. She spent many hours in their company and learned stories about the Dreamtime. She was very self-assured and adventurous, joining them in a variety of childhood activities.

While training as a nurse, she contracted a mysterious disease, "The Seven Plagues", that had killed many others and that resulted in one of her lungs being removed. She also became paralysed and totally blind.

During a year's convalescence, her sight and movement returned but she still tired very easily. Perhaps some of her intense empathy with the sick resulted from her own suffering. Even after returning to her training, it took several years until she felt fully recovered.

Her first nursing appointment was to the Point McLeay Mission. This fulfilled three desires of hers at that time: to be a missionary; to renew her friendships with the Aborigines among whom she had been raised; and to heal people using her nursing skills. Sometimes these skills did not seem enough and she occasionally placed her hands on people and prayed for them. It seemed that when she prayed like this some were healed supernaturally, especially among the Aborigines. They proclaimed she had "golden hands" and would seek her out to minister to them. Her bonds with them were strengthened.

The time was coming for her to expand her horizons beyond the locality of her childhood.

On holiday, she met Rosetta Flynn, sister of the famous John Flynn and perhaps his most vocal supporter. Ruth was fascinated by the stories Rosetta told and sensed that the AIM would continue her calling both to be a missionary and to heal people. She applied and was appointed to serve at Maranboy in the Northern Territory in 1930. There was an urgency about this appointment because both the incumbent Sisters were malaria-stricken themselves while trying to treat a general outbreak of the dreaded disease in the vicinity.

Sister Ruth and her companion, Sister Elizabeth Magaard, sailed to Darwin in the ss *Malabar*. The *Northern Territory Times* had this to say about them:

> The two new Sisters for the Maranboy Hostel carry with them the very kindly wishes from the ss *Malabar*. The stewardess fell seriously ill soon after leaving Brisbane and as soon as they heard of this the two Sisters volunteered to nurse her and spent practically all their time attending to the invalid. As they were the only two unmarried young ladies on board they were naturally much in request among the other sex; but the sick stewardess was of much more importance to them than any male passenger... So when they take up their work at Maranboy it will be with the kindly thoughts of all who know of their valuable services which undoubtedly saved the life of the stewardess of the *Malabar*.

From the moment the Sisters arrived at Penola Home in the tinfields of Maranboy, they found themselves working frantically. There had been a further outbreak of malaria following heavy rains and flooding. Patients streamed in from isolated areas several hundreds of kilometres away in all directions. The inundation of patients and the urgency of cases were such that Ruth wrote to the AIM saying it was impossible to estimate the number of patients they had treated.

One of the isolated communities worst hit was Mataranka, and Ruth and Elizabeth came to know the constables who served there. One of them, Ted Heathcock, came to Maranboy to ensure there was an airstrip suitable for a Flying Doctor aeroplane to use. After a period of courting, Ruth became engaged to Ted Heathcock and Elizabeth to Constable Frank Sheriden.

But all was not well at Maranboy with the hospital. The vituperative and paranoid Doctor Cook, famous for his arrogance, closed down Penola Home despite its 15 years of wonderful service and obvious value to the wider community. He was a domineering man and resented any medical facility over which he did not have total control, despite it leaving a community that included forty-three miners stranded a long way from help. The residents were furious and held meetings to voice their disapproval. One Territorian newspaper inferred that Cook considered himself to occupy "some position between His Majesty the King and the Creator".

Despite all the outrage, Penola Home was closed by Cook, thereby leaving Ruth and Elizabeth free to marry their beloveds. It is now that we see the brilliance of Flynn's strategy in employing nurses with commitment to his vision—Sister Ruth determined to set up her own nursing service along AIM lines at Mataranka and offer her services free of charge, just as the AIM did. She wrote to Flynn and asked to be given the AIM library books from Penola Home for distribution amongst the lonely pioneers. Flynn was delighted and agreed at once. At Mataranka, Ted had built a little library next to her new dispensary and the books found good use, especially as there were sixty unemployed men in the district.

Ted Heathcock, sixteen years Ruth's senior, was a most unusual man for those rough times. An Englishman, he was almost genteel in his approach to life. He was tall, strong and square-jawed, impressive and authoritative, yet he could be very gentle and doted on Ruth. Perhaps surprisingly, he shared her compassion for the suffering and disadvantaged. Throughout their marriage he gave her total support in her work as a nurse and had a profound respect for her unusual capabilities and special gifts.

It was at Mataranka that Ruth became aware of leprosy, that dread disease feared since biblical times. She found Aborigines with suppurating sores, easy to confuse with yaws in the early stages, but who had lost sensation in their limbs. One man had kicked skin and chunks of flesh off his foot, but appeared to suffer no pain. Others had skin rashes but did not scratch them or feel discomfort. A woman had burnt her hand dreadfully in a fire but discounted it. Ruth was shocked at the ravages this leprosy was visiting on its sufferers and began a lifelong service to lepers.

The couple was soon transferred to the very isolated Roper Bar. Ruth was convinced that her nursing must continue. Several times she was flown in flimsy aircraft to tend to the very sick when no doctor was available and her reputation as an outstanding nurse grew. Once Ted had his eye injured and there were long splinters of wood within the eyeball. With prayer and prompt action the eye was saved and even the doctor said it had been a miracle.

At Roper Bar, she established good relationships with local Aborigines, whom she nursed and with whom she had a real affinity.

As they began to trust her more, the Aborigines brought to Ruth those suffering with leprosy. They pleaded with her not to identify them because it would necessitate removal to the government leprosarium at Channel Island near Darwin. The Aborigines were terrified of this because they were not allowed to return home from there unless clear of all symptoms for two years, something that seldom happened with the treatments used in that era. Some tried to hide their condition, for example by covering the suppurating sores with a mixture of fat and ash or soil, resulting in a filthy mess. She was shocked at the large numbers involved and wondered where they were all hiding. Answers to her enquiries were evasive, but she deduced that the lepers were hiding in Arnhem Land, perhaps amongst the rocks and crags of a strange eroded landscape known to whites as the "Ruined City" or sometimes the "Lost City". She asked whether she could go out to see them in order to help them?

Her enquiries finally resulted in a mystical response from the Aborigines. Ted was away on patrol when nine, stark-naked tribal elders paid her an unexpected visit. Her Aboriginal housemaid was shocked and hid herself, terrified, in the kitchen cupboard. Ruth, though, realised something very important was about to happen and serenely greeted them. They surrounded her and wordlessly examined her ears, eyes, hands and feet, and finally her footprint. She humbly submitted to this examination and wondered what would happen next. They left without speaking to her, but they talked among themselves as they departed. Her maid was listening from inside the cupboard and told Ruth the men had determined that she had belonged to their tribe "in the Dreamtime". This conclusion opened the way for her to be allowed to visit the Ruined City to help the lepers there.

Subsequently the Aboriginal women taught her the language of the Alawar people, and gave her a tribal name that meant "the snake that will not sink". On telling them she could not even swim, they led her down to the river and pushed her under—but she bobbed up like a cork. They seemed satisfied with this.

Later they took Ruth to the Ruined City. It comprised strange erosion features that towered as truncated columns like thousands of giant teeth. The main section covered 8 square kilometres and provided quite enough cover for many people to hide in successfully. Ruth discovered a number of the lepers there and tended them. Arrangements were made for ongoing treatment and for a depot at which supplies could be left because many of the lepers were undernourished.

Ruth and Ted were in a sticky situation. As a policeman, Ted was required to uphold the law and transport any lepers he came across to the leprosarium near Darwin. But he respected Ruth's special touch with these sufferers and believed they would benefit much more from her treatment. The lepers would feel betrayed and no longer come to her if he apprehended even one in the course of his duties. What should he do? It would be no good appealing to the Australian Government that had made the law in the first place. Taking an enormous step that could have threatened his career, he wrote to the League of Nations in Geneva appealing for help in the situation. Ruth helped him compose the arguments. The upshot was surprisingly positive and Ruth was given special permission to treat the lepers in their own area without fear of removal. This she did.

In part because of the Heathcocks' intervention, the draconian laws concerning the treatment of lepers in Australia were slowly changed.

Subsequently, Ruth and Ted supervised Kahlin Compound, the facility for mixed-race girls in Darwin. With her concern for leprosy in particular, Ruth was shocked at the overcrowding; forty-four girls shared thirty-three beds by doubling up while others slept on the floor. The Government provided only twelve spoons, which were shared to eat the daily stew. As a number of girls came from leprosy areas, the risks were high and many did develop the dreaded disease later.

The Heathcocks served at the leprosarium at Channel Island for a few months in 1934 as a stopgap measure between changes of staff. Ruth was distressed at the treatment and conditions there and felt especially pleased that she had never compromised but had kept lepers away from the facility. It broke her heart when the Government rounded up some of her pariah lepers in the Mataranka area, chained them to trees until ready to transport them, and then consigned them to Channel Island—because she knew what they would face in that awful facility. However, by then another transfer had taken the Heathcocks to Borroloola, on the McArthur River.

In the February of 1941 a message scribbled on bloodstained paper came for Ted. He was away giving evidence in a case in Darwin, so Ruth read it.

> Have shot myself accidentally. Think I am settled. Can you come out? Shot the bone in two above the knee. May bleed to death. Horace Foster.

Ruth asked to see the young Aboriginal lad who had brought the letter. He was "properly knock up" and asleep on the floor, having heroically carried the message more than fifty miles across flooded swamps and rivers swollen by the Big Wet. She treated him for exhaustion and exposure before questioning him. He explained that Foster's camp was on the Wearyan River near the Gulf, where the white bushman produced salt from saltpans. She asked how long had it taken to bring the "yabber stick" and was told "two days". She found out as much as she could from him about the locality and landing possibilities so that she could brief the Flying Doctor.

Ruth swung into action. She called the Flying Doctor at Cloncurry using the police transceiver. During that day alone, an incredible 28 centimetres of rain fell on Borroloola.

The Flying Doctor tried to land at Foster's camp but found conditions too soggy and dangerous. He called in to tell Ruth on his way back to Cloncurry. She was visibly upset, imagining the agonies Foster might be going through. The Flying Doctor promised to try again as soon as the weather cleared a little. But a mini-cyclone had blown up, lashing the region with high winds and torrents of rain.

Ruth knew that Foster needed help as soon as possible. Her compassionate nature always drove her and she spoke to a local white "hermit", Roger Jose, considered a very good bushman. His lived in an old corrugated-iron tank with a bough roof and holes in the sides to act as windows and a door. Jose often wore a tea cosy for a hat and a heavy coat "to keep out the hot air". His piercing eyes were framed by wrinkled, sunburnt skin and silvery, curling hair. Would he take her to Foster? This unusual man stroked his long grey beard thoughtfully. Harry Foster was a former resident of Borroloola and his wife and two children, Jim and Roslyn, had lived there. His family had been evacuated to Sydney because of the war. Jose had had many friendly discussions with Foster, who was a kindred spirit, both men loving good literature. How could Roger Jose leave his mate Foster to die alone? But it would be insanity to try and reach the injured man taking this nurse along also.

"We could not get to Foster unless we went down the river, then sailed across to his camp. In this weather it would be impossible."

"Please, please. Please let's try." Ruth knew all about the crocodiles, sharks and snakes, but was prepared to try anything.

Jose pondered the situation for a few moments more while Ruth continued pleading, then agreed to try. He explained that they would have to travel by dugout canoe and he would take his Aboriginal wife Maggie and her brother to help, as it would be an arduous journey.

A dugout is hewn from a single massive tree trunk and is strong. However, its barrel shape makes it notoriously unstable in the water and any sudden movements could easily overturn it. Ruth had to try to sit very still while the strong men paddled it smoothly down the racing McArthur River, the rain still teeming down. Any wriggling to try and get more comfortable could have capsized them and Ruth could not swim, so she sat very still.

The men were wary of floating, uprooted trees and pushed these away with a "big-fella waddy", and in the quieter waters the powerful surge of swivelling crocodiles threatened to tip them over several times.

On the occasions that they stopped to rest, Jose and Maggie scratched for bush tucker to supplement their meagre rations. They looked for roots, insects, reptiles and birds, but the stormy conditions discouraged their foraging.

After travelling almost a hundred kilometres down the swollen McArthur, camping overnight, they emerged into the turbulent Gulf waters, which were blown by strong squalls. The men put up a bag for a crude sail to make use of the powerful winds. The danger was now extreme as they passed the notorious sandbar and into the swell of the open water. Ruth was in peril as she could not stay afloat if they capsized and they were drifting a long way from the shore!

By now they were all wet, famished and exhausted, but a further 30 kilometres lay between them and the mouth of the Wearyan River.

The tiny party reached the mouth of the Wearyan River after three more heroic days and nights. Cautiously, wearily, they made their way some 10 kilometres up it until finding Foster's camp, arriving the eighth day after the accident.

Foster raised himself slightly on seeing them. "Thank God you've come!" he exclaimed, and then fell back, his huge walrus-style moustache quivering. He insisted on talking some more and Ruth could tell from his muffled voice and twitching that tetanus might have set in already.

Ruth had to steel herself not to display any emotion as she inspected the wound. The leg was horribly swollen and black patches showed gangrene was advanced. Only amputation by a skilled surgeon might save Foster's life, and even then the chances would not be good.

Another white bushman, a friend of Foster's, arrived by chance. He undertook to prepare the landing strip, which was on higher ground, and did so. Ruth consequently sent a messenger to McArthur River station asking them to forward a message by pedal wireless. In it she pleaded for the Flying Doctor to come because the rain had slackened somewhat and the landing strip would serve. She also set about giving palliative care to Foster: hot foments gave some relief from pain and she set the bones skilfully and gently using bamboo splints.

The Flying Doctor plane came the following day and circled the soggy airstrip warily, knowing that to land in those conditions might put further lives at risk. But, after some hesitation, the pilot put the plane down safely.

Within an hour of the Flying Doctor's arrival, Horace Foster died. Ruth comforted herself knowing that she had eased his passing considerably.

On return to Borroloola, Ruth wrote a gentle and caring letter to Foster's family, reassuring them that Horace's passing had been peaceful. She hardly mentioned her own journey to find him.

Years later her bravery was brought to the attention of the Administrator of the Northern Territory, who exclaimed that her journey was "one of the bravest acts I have heard of". In 1951 she was awarded the MBE, in large part because of her courageous rescue mission but also because of her sacrificial nursing services. Sadly, Roger Jose and the rest of the rescue party received no awards although they certainly deserved the recognition.

With the Second World War came shortages, the threat of invasion and the expectation of evacuation orders any day. Ruth and others made representations for lepers to be sent to the South for safety and proper care. As the Aborigines trusted her, she was asked if she would escort a trainload of lepers from Alice Springs to Adelaide for treatment. This she did gladly. During this period she cooperated briefly with another former AIM Sister in Elsie Jones (nee King), who was running the leprosarium on Channel Island and whom she had met previously. Elsie's extraordinary inner strength impressed her.

Ted died in 1943. Their marriage had been especially happy and Ruth was devastated at first, but then pulled herself together to find where next she could contribute.

For the remainder of the war, Ruth provided care for Aboriginal children in an Anglican hostel in Alice Springs. But when it came time, after hostilities had ended, for the lepers to return to the North, Ruth made sure she went back to Adelaide to collect them. She knew, because of her reputation among the lepers, that her presence would be reassuring for them, and it was.

Ruth returned to Adelaide and continued her nursing there for many years, earning a reputation as an outstanding midwife. Her local council named her Citizen of the Year in 1988.

Although having many friends and attracting media scrutiny from time to time, Ruth somehow retained her privacy.

Her life epitomised the qualities Flynn respected most: a self-sacrificing spirit, compassion, optimism, expertise, courage, humility, good humour and unyielding faith.

* * * *

One of the women who interested and impressed Ruth Heathcock as a kindred spirit was Elsie Jones, who had also served with the AIM in the Territory. Their paths had crossed a few times and the bonds they shared as compassionate, determined nurses meant there was a natural empathy. They were also both appalled at the treatment of lepers and determined to do something about it, but took different paths. Ruth set about trying to change the law while Elsie worked within the law at the leprosarium at Channel Island near Darwin, but changed how the lepers were treated there. Both approaches complemented one another.

Elsie was fifteen years Ruth's senior senior. In practical nursing terms this meant Elsie had served in the Great War while Ruth had been too young. Elsie had been with the Australian Infantry Forces at the military hospital at Salonika and later served in Egypt and on a hospital ship, floating quietly but with death and trauma all around. The primitive conditions and unspeakable suffering greatly upset the young nurse and she determined, come what may, she would "do something to help others in life".

Her Christian commitment attracted Elsie to the AIM with its motto of "For Christ and Continent". She joined up and was sent in 1922, with Sister Jean Gray, to Penola House at Maranboy.

When the Sisters arrived in Darwin they were given an SOS from Victoria River Downs station (VRD). It came from Mrs Graham, the wife of the manager; two men had already died there in an outbreak of malaria and her own husband was dangerously ill.

The Sisters were told that the previous year the managers of Wave Hill and Burnside stations had both died from malignant malaria, along with a number of other men. The outbreak this year had started even earlier and was already rampant. Help was imperative if lives were to be saved.

The need was urgent. The two nurses pondered what to do.

"I nursed malaria during the Great War. I'll volunteer to go and help until the situation is under control," Elsie proffered.

"What will Mr Flynn think?"

"I'll wire him to ask his permission."

This took a while because communications were difficult to the South from Darwin, but Flynn was immediately in agreement. He was planning to build an AIM nursing home at Victoria River Downs soon in any case. Sister Gray would proceed to Maranboy to hold the fort until Elsie could join her there.

By the time Elsie reached VRD twelve men had died in the area. The manager, Mr Graham, was still alive. She tended all who came to the homestead, using the wide verandas. But she also went out to where the men lay: "I nursed the men in the huts, I tended the sick who camped on the bank of the river and visited others up to 100 miles away."

Through nursing of the highest order, Elsie halted the fatalities and there were no more deaths from malaria. Both Flynn and the Grahams remarked on this dramatic change and gave the credit to Elsie's extraordinary dedication and skill. Even a decade later, *The Northern Times* remembered and commended her Herculean efforts during this crisis.

Meanwhile, there had been a change of plan. Sister Jean Gray was sent to help Elsie at VRD and two other nurses were found for Maranboy. But for six months Elsie had nursed alone.

At VRD, Jean and Elsie had to tend the sick as they found them, or on the homestead verandah, until Flynn managed to build a hospital for them just 200 metres from the homestead. He rushed ahead, and as Jean expressed it, "the hospital was built around our heads". They pleaded with Flynn not to enclose the upstairs verandah with gauze because, in those stifling conditions, they would "rather die of mosquitoes than from suffocation". But building in such a remote location was a slow business and the hospital was not finished until shortly before they left.

They fought epic battles that necessitated courage and dedication beyond the usual, particularly because the women sometimes had to travel to their patients and conditions were rough. One such occurred shortly after Jean's arrival. From Elsie's report early in 1923:

> I do not know if you read of the murder of two white men by blacks down on Sturt Creek. Last October mounted troopers were sent out to catch the murderer, "Banjo"; this they did. While Mounted Constables Hood and Henning were on their way back to Katherine and Darwin, Mr Hood was thrown from his horse and sustained a broken leg.
> They sent back to Wave Hill for a conveyance to bring the patient in to us. He was lying in the bush for two days

before they could start; you can imagine the heat and pests this time of the year would make things doubly uncomfortable.

After two days travelling through the boggy soil and rough limestone country the patient was suffering so much pain that he could not be brought any further, so the other trooper rode into Victoria River Downs for one of us.

It took the trooper two days to reach us. When he arrived it had rained two inches and he had to swim across the river to get to me. But during that night a further 247 points of rain fell and the river could not be crossed for three days. The manager lent me a buckboard. Then, on Sunday 17th December, the horses were forced to swim and I went across in a boat.

We went 17 miles the first day and it rained all the time; the roads were boggy and the creeks all bankers. We camped at Gordon Creek. I could not sleep that night. The water was pouring in everywhere and mosquitoes were in millions. I was glad to see daylight!

Next day it rained solidly. In fact, it rained so hard that we had to stop. We got out and stood against the buckboard. But we got there despite everything.

It was 8 p.m. at night when we arrived and I did get a welcome from my patient, for his leg was so painful. By this time the leg had been broken twelve days! I got a shock when I saw it. It was green and blue and a dreadful size. I had to wait until the swelling subsided before I could find the damage. Both bones were broken. I gave him an anaesthetic and set the leg. I really did not expect that the fracture would knit, so badly was it bruised.

Next day his mate left. I stayed with my patient for six weeks.

Finally I removed the splint. With general massage he was able eventually to get about on crutches and then on two sticks.

I was anxious to get him back to the station, so after seven weeks we decided to try our luck. The stockmen lent us horses and we rode back. We had no meat, it was so hot that things went bad, but we had bread and jam. That was the main thing. It took us two days but it was worth it all.

After a further two weeks, he went back on duty at Timber Creek and has felt no ill effects since.

Imagine the discomforts of nursing beside the track for seven weeks in the Wet with scant supplies. She did not mention it, but this vigil beside the track was over the Christmas season. Elsie King was an extraordinary nurse because she often went far beyond the call of duty in this way, to the edges of human endurance, in her efforts to "do something to help others".

Through all her traumas, Elsie maintained a positive outlook that was infectious. Sister Jean commended it when writing about living together in great isolation:

> If you don't watch yourself carefully, you will find yourself growing morbidly sensitive over little things. For this reason we tried to find as much work as possible to do. On mail days we read each other's letters and discussed every scrap of family news. A new frock or a piece of material was a sensation! But try how we might, every conversation would become exhausted and we would fall into long silences. Then Sister King would remark: "Just look at the trouble that policeman is having controlling traffic out there", and I would laugh—and the dog would bark at the sound of our voices, and everything perked up.

Victoria River Downs was at that time the largest cattle station in the world, comprising 33,000 square kilometres. There were around seventty men and two women on the station itself and many visitors. The two nurses were much sought after for company:

> Being on one of the main stock routes, ours was what you could describe as a floating population. Besides cases in hospital, we entertained all the wayfarers—the drover, the prospector, the mailman whose delivery round covered 7,600 miles, the chance adventurer and the stockmen of the station itself. All sojourned with us a day or two, and all expressed their amazement that any two women should ever come out to such loneliness and isolation. We never seemed to make them quite understand.

Unfortunately these stray characters too often were carriers of malaria and other harmful diseases.

Shortly before their term of service was completed, they occupied the new cottage hospital, named "Wimmera Home". To celebrate, despite lacking amenities, they held a grand Christmas dinner to which they invited the VRD community. It was a happy occasion. Soon the new hospital became the social centre of the region, a home from home, just as Flynn had intended.

Their first patient in the new facility was Sarah Feeney, who remembers the AIM Hospital on the banks of the Wickham River as "beautiful". It certainly must have seemed so as she dragged her way there, heavily pregnant:

> I got down in the gully and I was holding my tummy and said to my hubby, "Wait up a bit". He replied in a panic, "Come on!" Anyway, I struggled up to my feet. The Sisters were just going to bed when we got there and he yelled out, "Are you awake? Well, here's a job for you!"

The delivery was successful but the story did not end there. When the husband returned home their eldest child, Grace, made a "terrible to do" over the absence of her mother. By the next evening the father had had enough of trying to look after the three remaining children by himself, so took them in to the hospital as evidence that they needed Sarah's care back home. The Sisters told Sarah, "Don't go. You stop here and have a rest to get your strength up. You'll have four children to look after when you get home, so let him look after them until then."

But Grace would not return with her father, so the Sisters let her stay with her mother and new baby brother for the duration.

The husband returned every night for a fortnight and pleaded with Sarah to come home.

If the nurses' attitude seemed a little protective, consider the lifestyle of women out there. Here are Elsie's observations made regarding the life led by another wife:

> Her husband being head stockman is away most of the time, leaving her alone for weeks at a time, so you can imagine how lonely it is for her. She has had a lot of anxiety with her children. They have had frequent attacks of fever. There is no comfort whatever for her but she is one of those brave

bush women who through it all keeps smiling. She has a garden that she does herself. She also does the killing and cooking, besides looking after her family.

Meanwhile romance had bloomed between Elsie and a drover, Bob "Jack" Jones (Elsie used the name Bob while others commonly used Jack). As was the situation with Ruth and Ted Heathcock, Bob was, "One of the best and will help me to still carry on with the work, only in a more indirect way. I think we will be living a few miles from Katherine. He may take up land there."

Indeed, Elsie saw her role in a wider context than the AIM alone, as she explained to a Methodist Church congregation in Darwin—it was Flynn's vision to supply a nurse within 100 miles of every isolated family in Australia and she intended to become a small part of that.

The heroism these two nurses had displayed was lauded in Melbourne's *Argus*:

> In a land that breeds heroes and has place for none else, there is not a man who would not vote these women who watch and wait to succour wayfarers on the world's loneliest highway the greatest heroes of all.

Almost a decade later the Melbourne *Herald* still remembered Elsie's heroism and wrote a feature article about it on February 31st 1931.

In the years following her work at VRD, Elsie was to need all her grit and courage. Her life at Katherine was extraordinarily difficult. Not only did she carry the nursing load for the area free of charge, but she also helped Bob daily, and sometimes at night by lantern light, trying to eke a living from the land. This was tough, physical work—and she had two babies, Jack and Barbara, in the interim.

Finally Elsie's health collapsed and she was sent to Melbourne to recuperate. A journalist who interviewed her on arrival asked if she intended returning: "She replied emphatically, 'Too right!' In this reply can be seen her incredible pluck."

As soon as her health began to improve, she began champing at the bit to return and help Bob because the peanut crop was more than he could handle alone.

Unfortunately the sale price for peanuts fluctuated and some years it became not worth harvesting them at all.

Not surprisingly, the peanut venture proved a disaster in the long term and the Joneses were living below the poverty line for their last few years there. So, after ten years, they walked away from it, never to return to farming.

Meanwhile Bob hunted for work. Because of the Great Depression, there was little available. Elsie, as a nurse, was more employable and became Matron of the Home for mixed-race children at Pine Creek in the latter half of 1932. She also cared for all sick and injured in the environs on a voluntary basis, there being no hospital. Bob helped her at the Home and later in the transfer of children to the facility in Alice Springs, the Bungalow.

During 1933, Elsie was called urgently to help out at the Wimmera Home during an outbreak of malaria where, once again, her outstanding dedication and skill saved many lives.

Bob applied when a position came vacant at the Bungalow in 1934. He was chosen to be the Superintendent and Elsie was to be the Matron. They took up the positions from 1st June 1934.

There were 140 boys and girls of all ages at the Bungalow in 1934. Since there was no government hospital, Elsie nursed all the sick children within the facility itself. The children had been immunised for diphtheria but other immunisations were not available. It was impossible to prevent the spread of diseases in the cramped conditions—two children slept head-to-toe on each bed and the extras slept on the floor. In quick succession Elsie and Bob coped unaided with epidemics of measles and whooping cough. It upset Elsie greatly that two children died from whooping cough.

They remained grateful for the work and the regular government salary that accompanied it, but the environment was unhealthy and their two children developed acute trachoma. They were advised that Jack and Barbara could go blind were they to remain in the Alice. Consequently Bob and Elsie applied, as a team combination, for the positions advertised at the notorious leprosarium at Channel Island, which was 12 kilometres out from Darwin's wharf. Elsie was appointed Matron and Bob the Superintendent as from 1st February 1937. Would a leprosarium outside Darwin really be healthier than Jay Creek? The unlikely answer was a guarded "yes", but only as far as trachoma was concerned. Therefore an agreement was reached for the children to live in Darwin and not in the leprosarium at all, although they would visit frequently. It was not an ideal arrangement but the best the Joneses could broker at the time.

Elsie was especially pleased that the couple replacing them at the Bungalow were Bill and Ina McCoy, because the children there needed special care and attention. Ina (nee Pope) had been one of the first of Flynn's Sisters at the Alice Springs Hospital and had the reputation of being an outstanding nurse. On marrying Bill McCoy, she had continued her nursing, often voluntarily in the mould of Elsie and Ruth Heathcock. [Ina and Bill did sterling work with the unfortunate mixed-race children at the Bungalow until evacuation in March 1942. Nor did they desert their charges then. They were offered Balaklava Racecourse in South Australia and Bill went ahead and did his best to turn the old buildings into a reasonable holding centre. Ina struggled on alone cooking and caring for hundreds in Alice Springs because the confusion of war swelled numbers alarmingly, until joining Bill and the evacuees at Balaklava.]

Bob and Elsie had heard that the care of lepers on Channel Island left much to be desired. Fundamentally it was operating as a quarantine centre and the Government had scant interest in what happened to the poor unfortunates who lived there. Bored, without hope and depressed with little else to do but fish, the lepers were quarrelsome and unhappy. Cliques had formed, based partly on skin colour and racial background, and the white lepers were the royalty. When lepers died, it was recorded in a book and the soft earth was easy to dig for yet another unmarked grave. Soon there was little soft soil left for graves, the published mortality rate over ten years being 69 dead and buried on the island, out of 187 patients. Doctor Cook, by choosing Channel Island, had the distinction of running the only leprosy colony in the world where the inmates could not grow fresh fruit and vegetables for themselves because the soil was too poor. Not only would this have relieved boredom, it would have improved the diet, and healthy food was considered important to recovery. As it was, all food items were government rations that came out weekly by supply boat from Darwin. Another factor Doctor Cook had not considered was that at low tides the inmates could simply walk off the island, which a number did and then led the police a merry chase to recapture them while the community in Darwin panicked. Most were recaptured but some disappeared—fate unknown.

The whole situation was depressing and unacceptable for a couple as positive as Bob and Elsie. They quickly and prayerfully planned improvements.

Bob found an unused signal lamp in the stores. He was an ex-army signaller and taught several patients how to signal using Morse code. As there was no school on the island, they enjoyed the opportunity to learn something to relieve the boredom. The signals could be seen clearly at night from the police station near Government House on the Esplanade. Bob extended the lessons to other practical skills. He combined this with introducing discipline and the raising of standards of hygiene. By and large the inmates responded surprisingly well, probably because he was a caring and friendly person and many had not had anyone take much interest in them. Some of the whites seemed to resent his growing popularity, however, and deliberately upset the smooth running of the routines.

Elsie, meanwhile, was determined to raise the standard of care given. Leprosy requires constant monitoring and extensive bandaging. She could not cope alone so she trained girls who volunteered to become her nursing aides. Some became very proficient and took over the burden of the bandaging. Elsie applied for them to be paid for their work, but this was knocked back initially. She tried to kit them out in simple uniforms, though, and they were proud of the service they rendered and any bits of uniform they had. Over a period of time she provided each aide with a full, smart, white uniform.

Together Bob and Elsie devised other regular, unpaid duties like sweeping, cleaning, chopping and carting firewood, supervising supplies and general maintenance. They imbued these activities with commendation and respect and those who cooperated found the satisfaction of a job done well and the self-esteem this generated.

A few would not cooperate and caused problems. One woman in particular had been a prostitute in Darwin and had contracted the most contagious form of leprosy, but was filled with resentment at being consigned to an island where the men had little or no money. She was incorrigible and was always fomenting rebellion of one sort or another. She found a willing ally in one of the whites. As they both had criminal records and unserved sentences, an appeal was made for them to be put into jails instead. This was refused on the grounds that there were no jails capable of holding lepers without them being a health hazard to the other inmates. So these two knew they were above the law and soon what little money there was around was in the hands of the woman. This was ironic, as there was little to be done with it on Channel Island in any case.

Sexual liaisons produced some babies. Doctor Bruce Kirkland, a gentle and kind man, removed these from the island because of the dangers of infection. He took them to Bathurst Island Mission where they were cared for.

Despite these deep problems, conditions improved remarkably. As they had before, Bob and Elsie generated serenity and hope in the direst of circumstances. A later investigation, involving a great deal of oral testimony, revealed that the patients had almost universally happy memories of the era spent under the Joneses. For many it had been the best time of their pathetic lives.

In 1938 and quite out of the blue, Elsie was honoured by the King with an MBE for her services to nursing. The citation mentioned her exceptional work as Matron at Channel Island as well as her other contributions.

Not happy to leave the incorrigibles so dissatisfied, Elsie spoke with one white man who had been causing much of the trouble.

"What could I do that would make you a happier man?"

"Get me off this island."

"I would love to, but you know I can't do that until you are well. Is there nothing else?"

"Yeah. Look at you, you have glasses, you can read. What about me? I need glasses. Why can't I have any?"

Elsie took his request to heart and began to seek out ways and means. She managed to get spectacles for him and for some of the other lepers also. Furthermore, in 1940, she organised for a private dentist to come out and treat the patients. This provided great relief from discomfort for a number of them.

As the facility came under military control for the war effort, Bob and Elsie lobbied for other improvements. They won some important concessions. One was a small wage paid to the helpers on the island. These set about their duties with renewed vigour and the tone lifted still further.

Evacuation was offered to Bob and Elsie in 1941 because of the threat of a Japanese invasion. What about their lepers? Elsie put in very strong applications for them all to be evacuated as soon as possible—an invasion by sea of Darwin would put them directly in the line of attack. It was agreed that they would need to be taken South, but the organising of such a move presented many problems. For example, the military were not keen to use their vehicles and commercial shipping shunned the lepers. Although leprosy was not as contagious as most people imagined, it carried the stigma of centuries. Nor was the hesitation totally unjustified: the ship's captain who had transported some lepers from Western Australia to Channel Island went down with the dreadful disease afterwards.

Because there was hesitation regarding the evacuation of the lepers, Bob and Elsie decided to stay with their charges despite an invasion looking more likely every day. The lepers would be far less agitated if they were there when the moment to leave arrived and everything could be organised properly. To facilitate their decision, the Government allowed their two children to remain as boarders at Charters Towers until the situation at Channel Island had been resolved. Meanwhile Elsie contacted a number of experienced people she felt could help in the likely evacuation and transportation of lepers, Ruth Heathcock being one.

Early in 1942, Elsie found that she was becoming uncharacteristically tired during the day. She had various check-ups.

She was actually terminally ill but did not know it. Bob took her across to Darwin for yet another investigation on 19th February. They were in the hospital and rushed outside when the first bombs fell. Then they dived back inside and took shelter.

Chaos reigned in the hospital. Six bombs fell in the vicinity—windows were shattered, debris reigned down and all the buildings received some damage. Mercifully, there were no direct hits and no patients were seriously hurt but three staff were injured when thrown against a concrete wall by the blast of one of the bombs. Elsie at once offered her services but there were twenty or so nurses and doctors running around and she was not needed

Her urgent concern was for the lepers. Had the island been attacked? There was no way of communicating with it to find out.

She and Bob dashed down to the quay as soon as the "all-clear" siren sounded around 11 a.m. It appeared like a scene out of hell, with ships alight, the sea on fire in patches from burning oil and the harbour covered in a pall of smoke. One bomb had cut the wharf in two and scurrying ambulance-men told them twenty men had died in that blast alone. It was hard not to be distracted but they searched for their boat, only to discover that it had been one of those sunk.

Despite the confusion, they managed to return to the hospital among a growing stream of injured and traumatised Darwinites. There they found ambulances disgorging the dead as well as the living. They also eventually located the kindly Doctor Kirkland, who had been examining the corpses mounting up in the morgue. Frantically busy, carrying an enormous responsibility, he was not able to take them out right away to Channel Island but shared their concern. He promised he would do what he could as soon as possible, which turned out to be the following day.

Meanwhile on the island the lepers had had a spectacular view of the bombing and sinking of ships while remaining untouched themselves. While horrified, they realised they were not the target and did not panic.

Later that day some American seamen, some with serious injuries, came ashore at Channel Island. An officer commissioned morphia from the clinic although some of the sailors panicked at the thought that lepers had touched it. The Americans sheltered in the shade away from buildings and tended their own sick to avoid contact with the lepers. The officer was furious to discover there was no telephone or wireless link to Darwin, but the patients showed him their signalling lantern. That evening they used it to signal Darwin and a boat came around midnight to collect the stranded sailors.

Bob and Elsie, as part of the emergency measures, were authorised to start evacuating the island immediately. The day following the bombing, they went out with Doctor Bruce Kirkland. After excited reunions, they gathered everyone for a briefing. The doctor told the inmates that food in Darwin was short, that the enemy could land any day and that they were free to leave and go bush and hunt if they chose. Otherwise, they could be transferred to the government Quarantine Station on the mainland, or even choose to stay on the Island and take their chances there. Bob and Elsie then began supervising an orderly pack-up and departure and went with the group choosing to go to the Quarantine Centre.

Chaos still reigned in Darwin, and at the overcrowded Quarantine Centre as well. The lepers were told they could make their own way back to their home regions or board the train in the special "lepers coaches" provided for them. Elsie went on this train and wished each one luck as they alighted along the journey, some returning to the cattle stations or buffalo-shooting camps they had originally come from. A holding centre was provided in Alice Springs for those lepers remaining who wished to be transported further south.

Elsie herself, far from well, left the train at Tenant Creek and went to stay with friends, George and Doris Easy, at Rockhampton Downs, hoping to recover strength quickly so that she could help further with the evacuations.

The sixty who chose to walk off the island and go bush found themselves, in the main, too weak to hunt effectively, so had to fend for themselves in other ways. They divided into three groups. One group camped upstream from an Army camp and cadged food without their leprosy being disclosed, another lived off the food the younger women earned on a Darwin beach by bartering their favours, while the third group hid out near Claravale cattle station and made contact with the Aboriginal stockmen, who fed them clandestinely.

By April it was clear the Japanese invasion was not imminent and someone began to worry about contamination of the community by the released lepers. The solution was typically simplistic; bring them all back to Channel Island, apart from those still in government care down South, and then think again. Consequently, the lepers were hunted down heavy-handedly. Some were arrested and incarcerated in gaols and even in chains until special "leprosy trucks" could be sent out for them. By the end of May all the white and mixed-race patients had been accounted for, as had the majority of the Aborigines, but some had died and others had vanished.

While this was going on, Elsie had not recovered. When she suffered acute blood loss on 10th March, the Flying Doctor was called for. The RFDS plane was fully occupied doing surveillance work along the coast in expectation of another Japanese attack. An alternative arrangement was made, for Doctor Walter Straede from Tennant Creek to go to her aid by car. He and his wife, with their dog, happily set out to do this. However, being recent arrivals and not knowing the dangers, they neglected to prepare properly and refused the offer of an escort from the police. When they had not arrived by the following day a search was organised.

George Easy drove while his son, Ron, a fifteen-year-old, tracked the missing vehicle. They found where it had left the recognised route. Eventually they saw it broken down ahead of them. However, the doctor and wife were neither sheltering in it nor under nearby shade trees. George opened the bonnet and discovered a broken fuel pipe. He also checked the radiator and found it full of potable water. They could see the footprints of the missing couple but it was getting dark and it was not possible to do more that evening. Fearing the worst in those furnace conditions, they returned home and assembled a party to start again at first light, but this time without Ron as they wanted to protect the teenager from a harrowing experience.

Within hours the search party found the dehydrated bodies of the doctor and his wife, lying where they had fallen in the merciless sun.

Elsie's condition deteriorated further and she was flown out by the RFDS as an emergency. She died in the Brisbane General Hospital on 17th May, aged only 54 years, of peritonitis arising from a bleeding duodenal ulcer.

Elsie died having fulfilled her goal, "to do something for others". And in some ways her work on Channel Island lived on after her to the benefit of the lepers there. The nursing assistants, in distinctive white uniforms and now paid for their efforts, tended the other lepers very well throughout the war. The tradition of being a caring community also survived to some extent, at least until the facility was closed for good in 1955, unmourned because it had been unsuitable from the beginning. A new and better facility was provided at East Arm Settlement.

In recent times, leprosy has become more easily controlled using modern drugs.

In Elsie King and Ruth Heathcock, southern girls sent there by Flynn, the Territory has two heroes of whom all Australia can be proud.

Heroic nursing captured and deserved most attention up to the Second World War, but other women had always played a less prominent but none-the-less vital role in Flynn's work. His wife, Jean, typified their input and we learn a little about her and others in the next chapter.

11

They Also Served—Jean Flynn and Others

Throughout Flynn's ministry women played a pivotal role. Heroic nursing captured the imagination but women were unsung heroines in other support roles: raising money, packing books and other items as part of Office Teams (OTs), writing letters of encouragement and helping with menial tasks in AIM centres, manning the wireless on cattle stations and acting as hard-working companions to nurses at cottage hospitals.

Jean Baird joined the busy Sydney Office Team in 1922. She was immediately impressed by the kindness of her boss, Flynn himself, who arranged theatre parties for the voluntary workers and often surprised them with little gifts to thank them. He basically left the running of his headquarters to them.

One of the most important support roles in the AIM was that of General Secretary, who had to carry a tremendous load with Flynn often "on the wallaby". Jean Baird fulfilled this wonderfully well from 1926. Intelligent and tactful, she undertook many of Flynn's delicate negotiations for him.

Jean married John Flynn in May 1932, when he was fifty-one and she in her late thirties. Quiet, discreet, reserved, efficient and fiercely loyal, she made him an ideal wife.

Flynn took her on a trip with him later that year to a number of places in the AIM field. She had never visited these but had written letters to supporters and nurses serving in them. She was tremendously excited to be going.

The Flynns spent several months touring. Both still worked, she at her secretarial duties and taking minutes of meetings, sometimes late into the night. Flynn attended many meetings. Sometimes his duties separated them:

> That night at midnight Jack departed for Townsville. [John was fondly called "Jack" by the new bride, and by her

alone.] The old goods train was his only way of doing it, so much to our regret, off he went. It would be a wretched trip, with no conveniences, but poor Jack never studies his own comfort and never complains about the hardships of his lot; his life is absolutely given to the great cause of relieving the isolation and medical worries of the bush, and no hardships to himself will make him pause.

A letter came from Jack this morning. Says the Perth folk warn him that they will not let him depart until he exhibits me.

We were there as they put the steps up for the passengers to descend. It was great to see Jack again.

She had a sense of the ridiculous and her letters are peppered with amusing observations:

Thursday afternoon the ladies of the town were invited here, and it was evidently an occasion, for it was the third time this year (being now November) that one good lady had worn her teeth! Sadly they have now been lost, having been carried in her pocket while picking peas, so I arrived only just in time.

At Oodnadatta, "up the road" means anywhere between there and Darwin, and "down the road" is along the track to Adelaide. Our Padre asked at the hotel for a man. "Oh, he's up the road," came the reply, so he sat down to wait. After two or three hours he went and asked our Sister, when he was advised that the man for whom he had been waiting had left Alice Springs the day before and would not be down for a week. [The Sisters had a transceiver and presumably knew that fact through wireless chatter.]

One beauty spot in Oodnadatta is "Angle Pole", where the telegraph line takes a turn from miles of running dead straight. The children at school were asked on a geography examination paper to name the poles. Some answered, "North, South and Angle".

One station man along the line informed us that they never mind the day they arrive in Alice, so long as they get there in the right week. And certainly nobody seems to hurry, either railway official or travelling passenger.

Perhaps her greatest thrill came from experiencing the outback for the first time. Her correspondence brims over with her enjoyment:

> Mr Lithgow [Methodist Missionary] selected for his camp bed the centre of the road, which seemed a rather risky spot, but nothing passed by. In the distance we could hear a camel bell, and next morning the birds sang gloriously in the trees. Our walls consisted of huge clumps of spinifex [spiny grass]. It was a great experience to be sleeping out under the stars in the centre of Australia, and we revelled in it.
>
> One interesting episode on the trip was the news that one of the men at our camp fire the night before would leave the AIM books he had finished with in the middle of the road some two miles out of Winnecke, because he was picking up a new supply. We kept a look out for the books, but there was no need as they spoke for themselves some time before we got up to them.

This quaint phrase "spoke for themselves" denoted how obvious the books were sitting in the middle of the barren road.

> There were six riverbeds to cross. As these consist of sand, with no water, you have to let the air out of the tyres every time you cross, and pump them up again on the other side.
>
> The journey up was interesting to me from beginning to end. Besides the novelty of it all, it told tales of past AIMers, travelling up and down under varied conditions. In the wee small hours of the first morning [at Alice Springs], Sister Nance Inglis arrived with a glorious bunch of wildflowers for me.

Jean modelled the role of a totally supportive and self-sacrificing wife for the superintendent of the AIM. During this time she made friends with Meg McKay, who was to succeed her in this role. Meg, who was also a nurse, had other special contributions to make, and her unusual biography is recorded in Volume II.

It was not only women in the AIM who had a part to play in the Mantle of Safety. As illustrated by Jeannie Gunn and Jessie Litchfield, pioneering women had a vital role also. For a start, their compassion made them carers, midwives and nurses—though unqualified. Secondly, if wholesome family life were to be established in the outback, they would have to be the prime movers. Flynn wanted to network them into his plans and always sought their support. So he visited homesteads and spent long hours helping the women with mundanities that otherwise could discourage them—like repairing clocks and kitchen implements and teaching the children their correspondence courses to give the mother a break. While there he would speak of nursing homes within 100 miles of every outpost and of Flying Doctors to release women of the nagging fear of illness or accident occurring within the family. Hundreds of outback women converted to his ideas.

Life, of course, was difficult for women in the bush, and Flynn often told this anecdote to illustrate how the Flying Doctor could help. Using Flynn's own words:

> Living on a lonely property in the far outback was a man, his wife and a station hand.
> The wife became ill—so ill, that she was nigh unto death. There was no telephone on the property, so the husband had to drive ten miles to the nearest phone. By good luck, he managed to contact the Flying Doctor, who said:
> "Yes, I will come. Have you an airstrip at the homestead?"
> "Yes, but it has been raining and it is under water."
> "Well, have you a ridge?"
> "Yes, some distance away."
> "Set to and clear all the trees off, then take the stumps out to make a runway. When that's done, contact me."
> So the husband motored the ten miles home and he and his man worked like beavers, cutting down trees and taking out stumps and making a level runway. When this was done, he drove the ten miles to the telephone and contacted the Flying Doctor.
> "I'll come right away," said the doctor. "Carry the patient there, then light a fire and on it put old motor tyres to make a black smoke as a signal to guide me to the spot."
> "I haven't any old motor tyres," said the distraught husband. "The only tyres I have are on the car." These, of course, were very valuable to him because they were difficult and expensive to obtain.
> "Well, use them," said the doctor.

Back at the homestead, the men made a stretcher on which they placed the uncomplaining woman. Because it was a long distance and he was afraid he might let the poles slip, his wife being a large woman, the husband fastened himself to them with a horse's harness.

Arriving at the airstrip, they gently laid the wife on the ground and prepared to light the fire. When it was blazing, the husband put on the first tyre from his car. Great black smoke billowed up into the sky, but not a sight was there of the plane. When that had died down, he put the second tyre on the fire. Again the black smoke signal, but not a sign of the plane.

When they came to putting the last tyre on the fire, they did so with a prayer and a hope, for life and death lay in the balance. Black smoke billowed up into the clear sky, thick and signalling.

To their joy, in the far distant sky they perceived a tiny speck, that grew bigger and bigger—the Flying Doctor! Their prayers and hopes had been answered.

The pilot landed the plane safely on the improvised airstrip; the doctor, helped by the men, loaded the woman into the plane and off they flew to a hospital several hundred miles away.

In three months time the wife returned to her home and husband, healed and grateful from the bottom of her heart to the Flying Doctor and to the mercy of God.

One might wonder why women were there in the first place, when life was so rugged. Ruth Paynter suggests:

> Of course it is her support and love of her husband and her love of the bush. The surroundings; the myall, mulga and gum trees, the beautiful coloured landscape and gems, the songs of the birds, the brilliant sunsets and clear starry nights, the peace and quiet, and memories—are all part of her life. Then again, the loneliness of a big city frightens her and the security of her home over many years prevents her from leaving although she is getting old.

But Flynn soon brought changes to the role of the woman on the land. Besides home duties and helping with the muster or the branding, she adopted the daily use of the transceiver because her husband was generally out of the house.

As time went on, women in the outback learned how to cooperate with doctors and nurses, often over great distances. More often than not they had to describe to the doctor the symptoms of an illness or the nature of accident injuries, and then administer medicine prescribed via radio or render first aid. At this they became adept, using certain guidelines provided by the Service.

They became the guardians of the medicine chests and the dispensers of medicines, following the Flying Doctor's instructions. These chests eventually held more than 100 items of drugs, other medication and first aid equipment, as well as a St John's *First Aid Manual* and a simple anatomical chart. Asterisks marked some of the items and indicated: "Use only on doctor's orders". Others were specifics, such as aspirin or iodine. It was thus possible to administer minor first aid or treat simple complaints with the help of the medicine chest without consulting the Flying Doctor. One of the suggestions in the directions for use was amusing: "If you *must* use the scissors for sewing, be sure to put them back!"

In emergencies, the doctor could give complex wound dressing instructions and even tell the caller how to use a hypodermic syringe for injecting particular drugs. The women then became the hands and eyes of the doctor so far away, but always looked to the Flying Doctor for affirmation. The first RFDS pilot, Arthur Affleck, told a funny story along those lines when he was mistaken for the Flying Doctor by Mrs McCarthy at Newcastle Waters, but was urged to play along by a local so as not to hurt her feelings. He got more than he had bargained for because she led him immediately to a woman who had just given birth to a baby.

While he watched anxiously, she took the baby from the mother, placed it on the table and proceeded to unwind yards of flannel from around its tummy, saying: "There you are, doctor, would you be having a look to see if I fixed up the little feller right and proper?"

Going right up to the table, the pilot peered down at the infant's navel, touched his tummy gently a couple of times and straightened up. Looking Mrs McCarthy fair and square in the eyes, he said truthfully, "I couldn't have done as well myself, Mrs McCarthy. You're a marvel."

And she was, as were hundreds of other women who acted as nurses in the absence of anyone else to do the work.

Frequently, while the men folk were away from the station, the women gave the radio operator details of prevailing weather and then tested the airfield. The usual method of testing the field was to drive a car or truck across the runway at speed.

Flynn always spoke highly of the natural abilities of women in the bush. One of his favourite anecdotes was that of the Territory's weatherman, who obeyed his wife's instruction to put the firewood under the tank stand, because she expected rain. He muttered "How can it rain with a temperature of 92 and a humidity of 40 per cent?" It poured with rain that night. When he questioned his wife, she explained, "I go by the ants. They build up around their nests when rain is on the way. You should take more notice of ants." And over the years the Flying Doctors also learned to respect the outback woman's common sense, helpfulness and ability to observe a patient keenly. As Flynn had hoped, they became junior partners in delivering health care to the Inlanders and provided a vital link in his Mantle of Safety.

And while this was developing, it remained up to the mothers of the bush to establish happy, successful families. An important part of this was in being the "Keeper of Traditions" and nurturing the family identity by remembering significant events like birthdays and first teeth, maintaining family correspondence and friendships, interrelating with teachers and schools.

One Patrol Padre recalled a graphic example of this vital skill when a bushman approached him with the question, "You don't remember me, do you?"

"No, sorry, I don't."

"Well, you baptised me."

That still didn't help the Padre, who had baptised dozens of babies, and this tall bearded man didn't remind him of any of them.

"Well, actually, the truth is, it was my mother's breast you baptised."

Suddenly he remembered! It had been on his first patrol as a young and shy minister. The baptism had taken place inside the homestead, but the baby had started to yell and scream. Undaunted, the mother had whipped out a breast to console her child and quieten him. This had worked but totally disoriented the young padre, who blushed and did not know where to look. As a result he missed the baby's head with his first attempt at sprinkling.

"Hoi. You've just baptised my breast!" the mother had exclaimed.

His second attempt was successful, but the story within her family that a Patrol Padre had baptised her breast became part of that family's tradition.

"We are that distinctive family in this universe whose mother's breast was baptised."

Flynn, a great champion of family traditions, loved stories like this.

Our final biography in this volume anticipates a new era. Women were about to move beyond the realm of heroic nursing and into other spheres of professional service. Doctor Jean White, the world's first woman Flying Doctor, was to blaze this new track.

12

Flynn's First Woman Flying Doctor—
Jean White

Flynn had a problem, a very serious problem. His dreams for a Flying Doctor network that would provide a Mantle of Safety over the Australian bush were in danger of being scuttled by a politician, E. M. Hanlon. This man was Minister for Health in Queensland and in 1935 announced a grandiose government initiative to remove government doctors from small outback towns and to replace them with cover by government Flying Doctors instead. This would solve his difficulty in finding doctors prepared to serve in the bush because one Flying Doctor could replace a number of resident doctors. It sounded good on paper, but Flynn was outraged—he had developed Flying Doctors to supplement normal medical services, not to replace them. Growing families needed a doctor available at all times wherever possible, not just to be flown out when there was an emergency. Even private practitioners would not be tempted to settle outback if the Government established coverage by a Flying Doctor and the small Inland hospitals would wither on the vine. Flynn believed bush communities needed resident health care before families would settle with confidence. "Mr Hanlon wants our pioneers to remain as pioneers always and our frontiers to be inhospitable to young families," he thundered. "Rather than misusing public funds, the money should be used to improve medical facilities in the bush and to give better incentives for doctors to practise there." He wrote this and many other arguments to Hanlon, screeds and screeds, but he was ignored and the Government proceeded with its plans.

Next, Hanlon blithely suggested the first government base could be at Cloncurry, from where Flynn's own Flying Doctor Base, the only one in Queensland, operated. After all, Flynn had proved how successful a Flying Doctor Base could be in Cloncurry. This was an unsubtle attempt to take over Flynn's

Flying Doctor scheme in its entirety in Queensland and Hanlon announced to the press that he would build a smart new hospital there and have three Flying Doctors on staff with two aeroplanes to service the outlying areas. This flamboyant scheme dwarfed what Flynn could supply. Not surprisingly, financial support for Flynn's Base at Cloncurry fell away alarmingly—the public was not keen to support a private scheme if the Government was going to step in and take over.

But Cloncurry was Flynn's original base and the flagship for the Flying Doctor scheme. Its collapse would herald a crisis of confidence and other bases could fall.

Flynn did his sums and decided that even if Queensland did put together a tacky scheme for government Flying Doctors, it would prove to be too expensive and inefficient for the other States to follow suit. However, the public would not be made aware of the realities involved until it was too late. Meanwhile, Flynn's dream of bases networked into a national Mantle of Safety would be dead in the water because it depended on public support.

Worse still, he faced harsh criticism within the Presbyterian Church that spread and disaffected some members of the AIM itself. The criticism was that Flynn was "shoring up" the Cloncurry base and other Flying Doctor work with AIM funds that could better be spent doing straight "church work" elsewhere. Again, he agreed with these criticisms in principle and wanted to give the Cloncurry Base to the community to have and to operate, but he could not do so if it was collapsing because of a misguided government initiative. "For it to prosper, our baby must be healthy before we allow public adoption," he reasoned.

Flynn frenetically lobbied Queensland Government members, but with little success. Then he devised a "crackpot plan" which, like all of Flynn's plans, became more reasonable the further you dug into the detail. For most dreamers, the devil is in the detail. With Flynn, it was in the intricacies that he illustrated his special genius.

In essence, his plan was this: to at once set up another Flying Doctor Base at Normanton to service the Gulf country, a service that the Government had proclaimed it would provide eventually.

Would this not simply confirm how sensible the Government plans were? "Their projected costs are already pushing their commencement dates back and the press knows this," Flynn reasoned. "If we can show everyone that we can do it right now and at little cost to the public purse, because private enterprise is many times more efficient than their cumbersome machinations, we will have made a point no-one can ignore. And we will have put in a Flying Doctor to supplement medical services and not to replace them, so the bush will much prefer our effort. If the politicians don't get the message, their public will through the press, I'll make sure of that, and a loss of credibility will force them to change. Politicians cannot afford to act against their voters."

It was therefore a contorted approach. It relied heavily on Flynn being able to find significant funding for it very quickly at a time when uncertainty was hurting his financial support as it was.

As in so many other crises, the way forward opened up for Flynn step by step, as he began to put his ideas into practice. "God always supplies the rations and it will be no different this time," he told George Simpson.

One major step was a very large bequest that had been given by grazier J. S. Love for the work of the Flying Doctor Service. Flynn arranged to see Arthur Fadden, who administered the fund, in Brisbane, and managed to persuade him to provide sufficient funding to make a start almost immediately. He wrote later to Fadden, with whom he had become fast friends: "I think the time has come to strike hard, and immediately, to vindicate the value of non-political initiative in medical enterprise… [To do so] must eat up funds at a riotous pace. But fast fighting generally proves cheapest in the end. Thanks for making possible bigger dreams and greater victories."

This desperation to "'fight fast" to discredit Hanlon's cumbersome plans explains Flynn's aggressive financial forays at that time. Not only was he using the Love bequest but he was also dipping recklessly into reserve AIM funds. If this venture failed, his future as superintendent of the AIM could be forfeit. There was a very real chance of this as opposition to his "reckless" schemes grew within the church.

The next and vital hurdle was to sell the concept to the public. Unless it was popular with the media, Hanlon could still choose to ignore the new initiative. So the choice of the right Flying Doctor was crucial—someone personable and with a bit of flair to capture attention would be ideal. Flynn and Fred McKay went through the applications with particular care. Fred was involved because the new Flying Doctor would be operating in his patrol area and he would need to work closely with him, especially at the start until he was properly settled. Fred was always an astute judge of character and he penned his notes on each application. For example, one read: "I have had vast experience in surgery, radiology, midwifery and physiotherapy...." but Fred noted: "Have seen credentials of this man sent with an accompanying and laughable photograph of himself—a rolling stone!" Such a weather-beaten man simply would not do for the media attention they hoped to engender. They had to be particularly careful not to make a mistake in their appointment.

Enter Jean White. Her application showed she was in her early thirties, came from good pioneering stock and was familiar with life on the land. She had qualified at Melbourne University in 1929 and had had a good mix of experience since being a Resident Medical Officer in both Adelaide and Sydney. Besides good professional references, there was a ringing commendation from her minister, Reverend R. Macauley:

> Doctor White has a strong, independent and resourceful personality. She would carve out a job for herself anywhere. She has interests outside of medicine, particularly tennis, and has a tolerant and humorous outlook on life.

Through years of experience, Flynn rated each of her character traits very highly for successful service in the bush and was impressed. Fred, who was influential in the selection process, agreed that she was the most suitable applicant. She was appointed officially in April 1937.

Flynn orchestrated the media interviews and releases very cannily. It worked! The newspapers loved the romance of this smiling, fair-haired and attractive young woman who had never flown in an aeroplane to that point in time, yet was taking on Flying Doctor responsibility for over 165,000 square kilometres of the wildest and most remote Australian bush. The world's first woman Flying Doctor would be in a David and Goliath challenge and would have "the largest medical practice in the world".

Wanting to keep tight control over what the media reported, Flynn discouraged Jean White from giving personal interviews at this time. He supplied most of the material for the papers himself.

The public responded well to Flynn's new Flying Doctor scheme and the level of financial support that came in for it was gratifying. But could they pull it off?

Fred went up to the Gulf country ahead of Jean White. When she arrived, he introduced her to many of the people with whom she would be serving in her new positions as Medical Superintendent of Normanton and Croydon hospitals whilst also undertaking Flying Doctor duties.

When Flynn himself visited Cloncurry in July, Jean White had been on the job already since April. She and Fred both went to greet Flynn and also met Doctor George Simpson, Doctor Gordon Alberry, Jean Flynn, Meg and Maurie Anderson.

Right from the start, the young doctor impressed the Flynns with her unbridled enthusiasm for her work. Jean Flynn observed in one of her letters:

> The first to arrive was Doctor Jean White from Normanton. She was not given much breathing space, for there was a case at McKinlay that afternoon and she acted as Flying Doctor instead of Doctor Alberry, who was otherwise occupied. She seemed to thoroughly enjoy herself too... Doctor Jean had three medical cases by plane: the first to McKinlay, another to Urandangie and the third on Sunday, when she and Doctor Alberry flew to Kynuna for an operation. She revelled in the whole of it.

Jean White had a major worry, though, that she told them about. She was uncomfortable about the way certain things were done at the government hospital in Normanton and was feeling isolated because of her concerns. She anticipated trouble ahead. Jean Flynn noted:

> We were all staying together and it was pleasant. We had great old chats. Jean White was just thrilled through and through to be taking part in the AIM family gathering, for she finds it rather tough at times in Normanton and Croydon; there is nobody there she can open up to and feel safe. She made up for it here and talked and talked.

An unexpected event during that AIM gathering moved the young doctor deeply. In the Cloncurry Base radio station one evening they all gathered around and listened while Flynn spoke over the network, describing its history and purpose. When he had finished, callers wanting to thank him personally for all that he had achieved jammed the network. They called in from hundreds of miles to congratulate him and descriptions like "miracle" and "life-changing" moved Flynn and the others there to the core. The calls expressing commendation and gratitude went on and on and Flynn "grinned broadly most of the time with pure thrill". They had to call a halt at 11 p.m. because the Superintendent was jumping on a goods train to Townsville at midnight. It was all an outpouring of love and gratitude for what Flynn had achieved and confirmed to Jean White the value of what she was part of. She admitted later to tears, but said she was in good company.

Then it came time to leave. Jean Flynn observed with almost motherly concern:

> Yesterday morning Doctor Jean White returned to Normanton. We have grown fond of her in our short time together and shared good fellowship. There may be storms gathering where she is working.

Storms were gathering on several fronts and Jean was going to need all her equanimity because of the various traumas ahead.

The first storm in her service arose over racism. As a straightforward Christian, she took everyone as she found them and the racism displayed by certain staff in the government hospital at Normanton disturbed her. Especially upsetting were the mixed-race patients that wanted to be in the white wards but were consigned to the Aboriginal wards, where they felt unwelcome and did not want to go. Furthermore, her modern gynaecological techniques worried some of the women and complaints were made. On top of this, Jean was non-judgmental but nevertheless frank when diagnosing venereal diseases amongst the menfolk, which was quite common in that community at the time. Embarrassed, some of these men did not want her to examine them and others objected to being treated by a "sheila". All these issues caused conflict between her and the Matron and the Hospital Board.

Curtly, and without due process, the Hospital Board decided to "terminate Doctor White's appointment as Medical Superintendent of the Hospital". This was a bombshell and threatened all Flynn's plans and indeed the Mantle of Safety itself. It put Fred McKay and Flynn on the spot. The "visible success" they were seeking threatened to rebound on them as a very public failure because they had not considered the sociology of the region carefully enough when appointing a woman.

On a personal level, Fred was distressed by the unfair treatment Jean was receiving, but conversely she was calm and philosophical, saying to him: "I have done nothing wrong. If I had I would have reason to be upset. As it is, I'm sure I've adopted the correct stance and am not prepared to compromise." She was determined not to bend her Christian principles, as she saw the situation, and therefore compromise was not an option.

Fred contacted Flynn and said he believed the AIM should remove her and its ministry from Normanton.

Flynn disagreed and his wisdom ultimately prevailed. "We will not withdraw from the area, Fred. We will continue to serve the people of Normanton and build our bona fides there… Always look beyond next Christmas. Doctor White can continue her Flying Doctor work and also run the hospital at Croydon. She will have plenty of work to do, all of it most valuable."

So Fred called a public meeting. It was well attended. He explained that the AIM had originally responded to requests from the people of Normanton to send a doctor to them. As they were well aware, it was not easy finding good doctors to serve near the Gulf. The AIM had found them a fine doctor with excellent references, and her services had been given free of charge. He

201

added the AIM would continue its work in the Normanton area but that Doctor White's services would be withdrawn.

Happily, and to Flynn's great relief, the rejection Jean experienced at Normanton did not cause a stir in the press. The Gulf country was a bit inaccessible to reporters and so the drama passed virtually unnoticed.

Fred, throughout the time of uncertainty and also later, had ample opportunity to evaluate Jean White at work and she won his regard. He admired her commitment to the highest standards while maintaining a friendly sociability. Looking back some sixty years later, he remembered her fondly:

> She was a girl of open Christian faith and believed that her work was a ministry. I found her to be congenial, with a lovely smile, and very personable. She was blonde with fair skin and wore a hat and a blouse buttoned to the wrist to protect her against the sun. I remember her hands in particular; she had lovely hands. She dressed in jodhpurs that were long riding breeches, close-fitting from waist to ankle, because travelling in skirts in planes had its difficulties. I saw her in action often and considered her to be a very good doctor, as did most of her patients. She met the storms that came her way with a quiet spirit and a positive outlook.

Jean subsequently moved to Croydon, "Where," she wrote, "there are beautiful iron lamp-posts in neglected streets, a Chinese 'joss-house' that has fallen down but still has a beautiful bell, and a fine Church of England that was restored by Cuthbert, the 'Gold King', who has made two fortunes and is now opening up some of the old gold mines." In practice Croydon was a relic of the goldrushes of the 1870s and existed now mainly to service surrounding cattle stations. She lived in a room at the local hospital of which she was Medical Superintendent and, having a love of exercise, she walked the old streets and commented on the bush smells carried on the evening air in her letters.

Would the people of Croydon and surrounds also reject her? Quite the opposite proved to be the case; they showed touching gratitude and enormous enthusiasm for her services. She, in turn, took them to heart and her warm and open friendliness enabled many of the women to discuss with her their most intimate problems.

Jean was especially popular with young children of all races. She used to travel with little gifts for them and instead of dreading to see the doctor they looked forward to her clinics. The fond nickname "Santa Claus" was given to her and stuck locally.

Jean Flynn had felt a special concern for the young doctor when meeting her in July and was careful to maintain a regular personal correspondence with her. So when Fred asked her to help him transport bush children from the seaside near Brisbane back to Trekilano, she used the opportunity to meet with Doctor White again, to encourage her. She was relieved to find the young medico still very positive about her work and apparently unfazed by the difficulties she had experienced at Normanton.

Interviewed on return, Jean Flynn was quoted in the *Sydney Sun* of 5th October 1937:

> I went with Doctor Jean White, the first woman Flying Doctor, when she made her first trip with her own plane and her own pilot… Doctor White is a most bright personality. She went up there six months ago and is now stationed at Croydon… This wonderful woman is giving medical attention to an area of several hundred miles.

This article, and others like it, ensured the public perception of Jean White's work was very favourable. Steadily, the tide of opinion swung in Flynn's favour and away from Hanlon's impractical plans. This can be seen by a reversal of the downward trend and the money donated to the Flying Doctor work increased once more.

Although never having flown before accepting the position, Jean flew 70,000 kilometres during her first year alone! Her monthly reports back to headquarters in Sydney reveal she was extremely busy. Medical work included telephone and wireless consultations, normal doctor's duties within the hospital, clinic runs to homesteads, outlying camps and mission stations—and flights to emergency situations. A number of these mercy missions relieved great suffering and also saved lives. Most of her emergency calls involved accidents or serious tropical diseases, although one flight to the Mitchell River station and then to Cloncurry was to tend a pathetic case of an Aboriginal baby born with a cleft palate and hare-lip. This flight of compassion covered 2000 kilometres.

When Jean returned to Melbourne at the close of her first year to spend a brief vacation with her mother, the media caught up with her and a number of complimentary articles were written, one describing her as "young, golden-haired and vivacious". Some papers dubbed her the "Guardian Angel of the North" and the description stuck, making her officially one of Flynn's angels. Here are extracts from the *Melbourne Herald* of May 12th, 1938 that portray her work in detail and rather well:

> "I love the life and am looking forward to my return," Doctor White said before her departure from Melbourne this week. "I have my own 'plane, a Fox Moth. It has folding seats so that a stretcher can be accommodated comfortably if a patient requires moving to hospital...
>
> "There is always something of interest going on at the hospital," said Doctor White when asked how she spent her spare time. "I have plenty of books, and work which I took up with me is still lying untouched, so you can see I have plenty to occupy me.
>
> "It is not wise to go out during the hottest part of the day, but the evenings are ideal for walking. You in the South cannot imagine the beauty of the clear, starry nights with the heavy scent of frangipani in the air."
>
> Doctor White's work takes her among the Australian Aboriginals, and a gentle, almost motherly, note crept into her voice when she spoke of them. "I love them," she said. "They are splendid patients and so grateful for anything I do for them."
>
> The wet season, which lasts for about three months of the year, is one of the greatest drawbacks to Australia's Flying Doctors, for at present very few of the landing grounds are able to stand up to heavy rain without becoming boggy. However, with the help of the

Defence Department, improvements are steadily being made and now most homesteads have a reasonably good landing ground within a distance of five miles. [The Defence Department was gearing up for the approaching war].

Every precaution is taken to ensure safety in the air. Regulations regarding the use of the Qantas plane, which is overhauled every 25 flying hours, prohibit night flying, and Doctor White and her pilot are frequently at the aerodrome before dawn ready to make a start as soon as the instruments are visible. "Usually we prefer to follow the coast or a river as far as possible," she said, "but at times we have to detour to avoid storms. The pilot points out storm clouds to me and I quite enjoy our dodging them."

Doctor White spoke enthusiastically about the future of flying as a means of obtaining medical aid for people isolated from civilisation. She described the ordeal of transporting a patient over the bad roads of the outback and the comparative comfort and speed of air travel. "One man," she said, "living 60 miles away, cut his hand and decided to come to me for treatment. He left by car at 8 a.m. and reached me at 6 p.m., whereas I could have travelled the same distance comfortably in less than an hour."

Jean had said she enjoyed the thrill of dodging storms in the tiny Fox Moth biplane. Soon that thrill would turn into something much more sobering.

This was in the era just preceding the Second World War when women were struggling for professional recognition in a man's world. It was still a time of gallantry towards women. Despite this, some letters to the press questioned the wisdom of her work in the Gulf Country where the air was unstable and the conditions unpredictable. "If her plane ditches in the North, she'll be too soft to get out alive," was one view expressed.

The terrain made the chances of a fatal accident much more likely. Here, from a *Sydney Morning Herald* of early 1939, is a description of the country in which she worked:

> There are several nursing homes in the area, which is thickly populated with Aborigines, scarred with unfordable rivers, and, except in the more densely populated parts, has few roads worthy of the name. Parts of the coast are entirely isolated except for a ship which calls monthly. An Inland Patrol Padre patrols the Peninsula on horseback carrying on the work that was begun 25 years ago with camels, but the whole of the medical aid is achieved with the use of aeroplane and wireless.

Jean White was not oblivious to the fact that, were she to crash, the odds of locating her in the vast, empty regions were not good. And in her letters to her family, she admitted to extreme discomfort while bouncing around in a tiny aeroplane high above the rugged Gulf Country, although she quite enjoyed the thrill.

Balanced against these concerns was Jean's confidence in the bravery and sheer professionalism of her pilot, Captain Doug Tennant. He was known as a "good bush pilot", an epithet that denoted he operated with skill and common sense. Time and again he extricated them from tricky situations.

However, the day predicted by the "dismal Johnnies" finally came towards the end of January 1939 when the Flying Doctor aeroplane failed to arrive at Mitchell River Mission. For some reason, still unexplained, the lost aeroplane was not reported during the first two days it was missing.

Belatedly, Traeger's transceivers were put into operation. Had anyone seen the aeroplane? All cattle stations remotely near the intended flight path were alerted. No one had seen the plane since take-off. This may have been because most people had been sheltering indoors from the cyclonic storm that had whipped up and was still raging across the region.

Concern mounted as the hours passed without news. Surely a tiny aeroplane could not have survived such conditions? A crash must have occurred! The police and hospitals were alerted. Qantas began an immediate search along the flight path with Dragon and Fox Moth aircraft. They found nothing. The area of the search was widened to allow for violent winds blowing the lost plane off course. Fergus McMaster, one of the founders of

Qantas, and a pilot named Swaffield, who had a high regard for Jean as he had often taken her on Flying Doctor missions, flew search patterns. But as they looked down at the empty, green vastness below they were struck by the immensity of the task. But despite the unlikelihood of success, they flew hour after hour with hardly a break.

The Aboriginal people at Mitchell River station met together, sang hymns and prayed that their "medicine lady" might be found alive. Jean White's compassionate approach had endeared her to them. When there was a lull in the storm, they gathered in little knots under the mango trees and prayed further.

Soon the story broke in the media—Doctor Jean White was missing and her aeroplane had presumably crashed.

All Australia waited anxiously for news while the drama unfolded in the North.

* * * *

Jean had collected medicine bottles from Lotus Vale station and had visited various places on the Cape York Peninsula. It was Friday January 27th and the sky was clear and the weather calm when the Fox Moth lifted from the airstrip at Delta station, bound for the Mitchell River Mission.

Ever alert, Captain Doug Tennant had seen an ugly storm building ahead of them, so changed direction to fly around it. This used up valuable fuel. Then powerful north-west winds in the cyclone caused the storm to race back over their path. Soon their route to the Mission was cut off. He kept circling, waiting for the storm to moderate.

Now running short on fuel, he tried a desperate run into the storm to try and penetrate it and reach the Mission, but was tossed about violently by the winds. Visibility dropped to zero. He turned the plane and strong gusts spat them out. He was most relieved to escape the maelstrom in one piece.

The engine rattled and misfired, warning Tennant that his fuel was coming to an end.

"What was that, Doug?" Jean called out through the intercom, trying to hide her concern.

"Check your safety belt is tight. Our fuel is nearly finished. I will have to put her down soon." Tennant's eyes scoured the terrain as he spoke, looking desperately for a clearing on which to crash. The thick tree-cover gave little hope. This was mangrove and swamp country, heavily wooded and sparsely populated.

As their height dropped, Tennant saw the wide Mitchell River below them and noticed a sandy oasis in the expanse of water, Cocomungin Island. Here, at least, was hope, providing they could find a stretch of sand without trees or rocks.

Jean felt no fear, just mild apprehension, as they glided towards the island.

Tennant put the plane down as slowly as he dared. Any slower and the engine would have stalled. The ground still rushed up at them with frightening speed.

The wheels ran smoothly along the sand at first, a testament to the pilot's skill, but the rain had produced some soft patches. The wheels caught in one of these while they were still moving quickly, tipping the nose of the plane into the sand. Jean felt herself being lifted high, then turning right over and, finally, crashing down. The plane had dug its nose in, somersaulted and flipped onto its back.

The doctor found herself upside down and crushed under a weight of tangled gear: wireless equipment, medicine bottles, cases, tinned foods and potatoes. Her right arm was in great pain and she could not release her safety belt with her left hand alone. Was Tennant badly injured, perhaps killed? Her instincts were to do what she could to reach him, but her struggles only increased her pain. She was well and truly pinned down.

She stopped struggling for a few seconds to catch her breath. In the silence she heard noises above her. It was Tennant forcing open the cabin in order to reach her. Next thing he was tossing out the gear that was pressing down on her.

Once free, she was surprised how shaken she felt. Nevertheless, she managed to ask rather breathlessly, "Are you all right, Doug?"

"Yes, a bit battered, but otherwise fine. Your arm doesn't look too good to me."

"No, it's not." Her right arm hung limply. She examined it quickly using the fingers of her left hand.

"Can I do anything for it?"

"No thanks. It's not broken, just crushed. It will become mobile again in a while. Here, let me give you a check-up."

Tennant did not argue. Doctor White had always impressed him with her no-nonsense approach. He submitted to her medical examination.

When she was satisfied he was only bruised and had no broken bones or obvious internal injuries, she inquired, "What's our situation here?"

"That's a good question. The plane is out of commission, quite obviously, so we'd best sit tight until the storm has blown itself out. I'll set us up with a crude shelter, then radio out for help." Both were soaked through already and rivulets streamed down their faces and dripped from their fingertips, but the water was warm and exposure posed no immediate threat.

Jean discovered her right arm remained fairly useless as they rigged up a rough shelter using branches and a tarpaulin scavenged from the aeroplane.

"It will only have to last us a day or two so we needn't make it too fancy," Tennant observed.

Tennant removed the radio from the aeroplane and set it up by a tree. He hung the long aerial wire in the branches. It would not transmit. He turned the dial to "receive". Radio chatter came faintly through. He turned to "transmit" again, but that circuit was dead. He returned to the crude shelter to discuss their position with Jean.

"The radio was damaged in the crash and I can't repair it," he told her grimly. "We are some distance off our intended flight path, so it will take rescuers awhile to locate us, if at all."

They would need to settle down and wait for rescuers to come, so they returned to the upended aeroplane and dug around inside. They pulled out tins of sardines, a few tins of vegetables and a number of loose potatoes. "The bright side is that we have enough food to last us several days," Tennant observed, putting as good a spin on it as he could. "Providing I can find us fresh water to drink, I think we should sit tight and see what transpires. If they haven't found us by the time our food runs low, we'll try to walk out. I don't fancy that because there are very big crocs in the Mitchell, some of the biggest in the world, and also tangles of creeks and mangroves and thick bush between civilisation and us. Our best hope is that someone'll find us first."

Tennant went in search of potable water, the river being estuarine and too salty to drink. To his delight he found good, fresh water about three kilometres from the crash site. He also discovered the island to be bigger than he had supposed, though uninhabited.

When he returned to their makeshift camp dusk had arrived and with it swarms of ravenous mosquitoes. The two crash victims found themselves helpless against the hordes of stinging insects. By 11 p.m. their arms, legs and faces were swollen and they were desperate.

"I can't stand this anymore," Jean said. "Let's look in the plane for something to cover our heads with, even boxes or paper bags would help. I won't last the night with all the stings I'm getting."

They ransacked the cargo by moonlight, tearing open the parcels impatiently. Doctor White let out a squeal of delight. "Hey, look at this," she said, holding something aloft in triumph. It tumbled down from her hands and glowed a silvery white in the moonlight like a beautiful bridal veil—mosquito netting! The nets had been intended for Dunbar station. "How I thanked God when I saw those nets," she wrote later. She did not mean it flippantly.

They draped the nets over and around themselves as best they could and had relief from the relentless stinging for the first time in hours. Jean took a grim pleasure in the angry whining of the frustrated mosquitoes as they attacked the net time and again, but without success.

"What's that noise?" she asked Tennant later.

"Crocodiles thrashing around."

"Are we safe here?"

"We are far enough away from the riverbank, I think," was his laconic reply.

Saturday and Sunday passed. The cyclonic storm had abated and the skies were blue, but empty. It was especially frustrating to hear the radio messages exchanged between search parties out looking for them, as they were unable to transmit their position. Tennant began to think seriously about crossing the Mitchell and walking out.

Then, on the Monday, a plane droned overhead. They waved their arms and shouted, but failed to attract its attention.

"Damn, I thought they would have seen our crash. We must organise ourselves better to signal an aeroplane, if we are lucky enough for another to come close. I'll stack a fire to light when we hear one coming."

"Isn't the bush around here too wet for that?"

The next day they heard the plane before they saw it. Their frantic attempts to light the fire failed. Tennant then grabbed Jean's hand mirror and flashed it in the sun. They both stood in a clearing and Jean waved her left arm frenetically, her right being too tender.

The pilot, Swaffield, saw the flashes and dropped low to investigate. They now both waved madly. The pilot waggled the wings of the plane to show he had seen them, then banked and executed a wide circle before dropping rations and a message—they were to stay where they were and a rescue party would be sent out at once.

The rescue attempt was held up until Constable MacNaught was located. He was the man with the local knowledge needed to lead a party of men through the bush to Cocomungin Island. On arrival there, high tidal waters that teemed with salt-water crocodiles thwarted them. Undaunted, Constable MacNaught lashed together a raft for the crossing. Two Aboriginal searchers followed behind him, each bravely paddling on logs.

When part-way across, Constable MacNaught heard a yelling behind him. He swivelled to see a long dark shape gliding through the water towards the two Aborigines! He yelled out for them to change direction. The crocodile swirled in the water and headed towards MacNaught instead! Knowing an attack on the raft would tip him into the water, he raced back furiously towards the bank again. The crocodile hesitated when the water became very shallow. MacNaught leapt off and dragged the raft up to the land. When he had caught his breath sufficiently, he radioed a message to search headquarters to send out more men and equipment.

The following day a second party arrived that included Flying Doctor John Laver along with Fergus McMaster and others. Protected by guns, they and MacNaught made the crossing at low tide when attack by crocodiles was far less likely.

Jean and Doug first saw their rescuers at 8.30 a.m. on February 1st, a full five days since their crash.

After brief greetings and enquiries, Doctor Laver insisted on examining both Doug and Jean. He immobilised Jean's bruised arm in a plaster cast so that she would be able to walk out without too much pain. She told him sheepishly, "We've been too busy for me to notice it much until now." The party then turned back towards the river, needing to cross before the tide rose again.

All Australia celebrated their safe return.

Doctor Laver, after discussions with an exhausted Jean, wrote an interesting report to AIM headquarters. Among other things, he recommended the single-engine Fox Moth be replaced by a twin-engine Dragon. He was also critical of the particular wireless set used, which he stated had a reputation for unreliability, quoting no less an authority than Fergus McMaster. "It often requires coaxing to make it work properly and is too delicate to survive a crash". A more rugged, expensive and less temperamental set should be used. Flynn moved at once on both these suggestions.

Jean was not fazed by the accident and was flying again on a mercy mission within a few days. The drama of her accident and rescue brought favourable publicity, the *Sydney Morning Herald* reporting it on 6th February 1939 under the heading:

Guardian Angel of the Inland

> "Guardian Angel of the Gulf Country" is the term that has been applied to Doctor White… Most Australians were aware that a Flying Doctor named Jean White was doing some splendid humanitarian work in Northern

Queensland, but few were aware how hazardous and great was her work, how vast the territory she patrolled, until she and her pilot were reported missing.

The newspaper followed this introduction with the kind of human-interest article that gladdened Flynn's heart and widened support for his dreams.

The flashing of Jean's mirror that had caught the eye of the search pilot became folklore in the RFDS for a while, and we find Doctor Woods recommending isolated airstrips should use mirrors as a matter of course. In 1941 he formalised this unusual advice in instructions issued to homesteads: "Flash a good-sized mirror in the direction the plane is due to come. Your flashes will be visible 25 miles away".

How did Jean really feel about her work? She revealed this in an interview with a *Sydney Morning Herald* reporter. "I love the life and feel that I'm really accomplishing something," she enthused.

"And how do you survive the hot climate?"

"It is very hot but I don't find it unpleasant. The country is very dry except in the wet season, when the rivers run so high that settlers 50 miles away could not reach us. That is why the use of aeroplanes is so essential for our medical work."

"And what food do you eat?"

"We live in cattle country but we have to use goat's milk. It's really good. We've plenty of beef but we never see a sheep, so we eat goat. You have to acquire a taste for it. Our vegetables are tinned or dried, but we get fresh butter."

She certainly thrived on the life and lifestyle.

While her reports back to headquarters were terse and businesslike, masking much of the drama of her work, others wrote letters of appreciation that went into more detail. Flynn made sure to publish these in the press. Here is one such:

> Sir,—May I put before your readers some of the work done by the Aerial Inland Mission through the Flying Doctor. From December till April we are cut off from the world by flooded roads and cyclones in the Gulf. If serious sickness or accident happens, the Flying Doctor is our only hope.

> At the mission we have 300 Aboriginals, apart from the semi-wild nomads who come in when they are sick. The Flying Doctor has saved many of their lives and within the last month, the life of a white. Nearby stations can tell the same story of service to both white and black employees.
>
> We have had two cases of sickness among the white staff here in a month. In each, a wireless message was sent in the morning and the doctor was here by nightfall and removed the patients to hospital. The AIM has worked for all, without counting colour, creed or race.
>
> Doctor Jean White has charge of our district, and whenever she is within a hundred miles of the mission, comes on to see our sick Aboriginals. This is of the greatest value. We have no trained medical staff, only amateurs doing their best.
>
> The AIM has no red tape. A call is sent to them, and at once they answer it, if flying is at all possible. They never ask for payment, the service is freely given. Those who can give what they can afford as a donation, but such an enterprise as the AIM Flying Doctor Service, together with wireless and other heavy expenses, would render it impossible for a working-man or a mission, on behalf of its Aboriginals, to make adequate payment. Only by public support can this magnificent work be carried on.
>
> > Yours,
> > PHILIP SEYMOUR,
> > Chaplain, Mitchell River Mission.

Jean White's very evident success finally caused Hanlon's expensive plans to replace existing doctors with Flying Doctors to be abandoned. The plans were never officially withdrawn, for to do so would have lost too much face, but they were shelved quietly in August 1938 as "unworkable at present"—and thus Flynn, with Jean White's help, had won another vital battle for his beloved bush.

At the end of her contract, in August 1939, Jean returned to private practice in Melbourne. She kept ties with the AIM and supported Flynn's vision as a benefactor.

Jean White was among the throng of well-wishers at the opening of the John Flynn Church in Alice Springs in 1956. Still hale and hearty, she helped organise some of the outings to local features. At this time she was still in private practice in Melbourne.

Despite her warmth and charm, and attractive looks, Jean never married. She passed away in 1975.

* * * *

In some ways Jean White blazed a new track, proving that women could serve in the most difficult of outposts as professionals in capacities other than nurses. And the Second World War, that was soon to follow, would sweep aside the myth that women could not serve on a par with men.

Flynn would welcome, indeed embrace, this change in perception about the role of women as he had been ignoring the old clichés for decades already. Therefore it is fitting that his vision was about to be taken forward by a new breed of professional woman, building on the magnificent work done by the nurses at the outposts. The input of nurses would continue to be important after World War II, but alongside them in the outback would serve female pilots, Flying Doctors, Patrol Padres, dentists, vets, social workers, Flight Nurses and a variety of innovative educators led by Adelaide Miethke and her "School of the Air".

It was an era of exciting change. Flynn's visionary work was about to surge ahead. A new day was dawning and fresh pages were about to be written in the annals of women's achievements in the outback.

Flynn's Outback Angels Volume II.
Fulfilling the Vision, 1941–2001
Stories of women pilots, flying dentists, doctors, flight nurses, teachers and outback nurses.

RRP $25.95*

Secure your copy of Volume II now!

Part of the trilogy which includes:

Flynn's Outback Angels Volume I.
Casting the Mantle, 1901–WW II
Stories of pioneering women and Flynn's outback nurses in the first half of the twentieth century.

RRP $25.95*

John Flynn:
Of Flying Doctors and Frontier Faith

RRP $25.95*

SAVE! any two books $45.00*!

SAVE! any three books $65.00*!

Please send me the books indicated below:

John Flynn ____ copies; Volume I ____ copies; Volume II ____ copies

Name _____

Address _____

_____ State ____ Postcode ____ Phone (__) _____

I enclose my cheque/money order for $ _____ OR

(Please do not send cash by mail)

Please charge my Bankcard ☐ MasterCard ☐ Visa ☐

Card No. ____ / ____ / ____ Expiry Date ____ / ____

*All prices include GST. Please add $3.00 postage and handling

Signature _____

If you'd like to order other titles or need to add more information, please attach a separate sheet of paper to this form.

Post to: **Old Silvertail's Outback Books**
PO Box 1615, Rockhampton, QLD 4700 *OR* Phone, fax or email your order* to
Phone (07) 4923 2520, fax (07) 4923 2525, email d.myers@cqu.edu.au
*Don't forget your credit card details
When ordering, ask for our catalogue